Recipes
For
DIABETICS

by Billie Little with Penny L. Thorup

Preface by Gerson A. Jacobson, M.D.

Diabetes is a metabolic malfunction that affects an estimated four million Americans. Although potentially serious, it can, with proper medication and diet, be kept completely under control. Crucial to that control is diet.

When diabetes is diagnosed, the patient is given, by his doctor, a list of what foods he can eat, in what quantity, and at what intervals. Armed with this information and with various necessary charts and lists, he all too often sets forth to a diet of unremitting monotony. So time-consuming is it to extract from the standard cookbook recipe the information needed to calculate the diabetic's requirements that often a diabetic will rely upon but a few tested and measured dishes. This cookbook is written to change that. It is written to guide cooks in preparing and serving attractive, colorful, unusual, satisfying, and varied meals that conform to the individual dietetic needs of the diabetic —and that can be enjoyed by the non-diabetic as well!

Each recipe has been calculated to include the caloric content as well as the exchange-group breakdown for each measured individual serving. Each recipe has a simple system to

Continued on back flap

Recipes
For
DIABETICS

Recipes
For
DIABETICS

by Billie Little with Penny L. Thorup

GROSSET & DUNLAP, INC.
A NATIONAL GENERAL COMPANY
PUBLISHERS   NEW YORK

CONTENTS

ACKNOWLEDGEMENTS

So very many friends, relatives and diabetic patients have contributed their ideas and treasured recipes that we wish to give a special note of thanks to them and to the food companies, firms, newspapers, and magazines whose information appears in this book. We gratefully acknowledge the following permissions:

Alberto Culver Company, Melrose Park, Illinois 60160 (Sugartwin)
Campbell Soup Company, 375 Memorial Ave., Camden, New Jersey 08101
Cumberland Packing Co., 2 Cumberland St., Brooklyn, N. Y. 11205 (Sweet 'n Low Division)
Eli Lilly and Company, Indianapolis, Ind. 46206
Hollywood Foods, 340 Azusa Street, Los Angeles, California 90012 (Safflower Division)
Knox Gelatin Incorporated, Johnstown, N. Y. 12095
Lever Brothers, New York City, N. Y. 10022
Pillsbury Company, Minneapolis, Minn. 55402 (Sprinkle Sweet)
Plough, Incorporated, Memphis, Tennessee 38101 (Ril Sweet)
Spice Island Division, Leslie Foods, Inc., San Francisco, California 94133
Tillie Lewis Foods, Inc., Drawer J, Stockton, California 95201 (Low Calorie Foods)
U. S. Department of Agriculture, Washington, D. C.
U. S. Department of Health, Education and Welfare, Public Health Service, Washington, D. C.

SPECIAL THANKS TO: Mrs. Editha Carlson, Public Relations Division, Eli Lilly and Company, Indianapolis, Indiana, for her assistance and permission to use information contained in the many excellent booklets distributed by this fine company; to Mr. Frank Schubert of Tillie Lewis; to Dr. Gerson A. Jacobson; the Public Health Service and other sources which have been used; to Marie Slavens our typist for patiently wading through our notes; and last, but not least—Jonathan Bartlett, our faithful and untiring editor.

Additional information on medication, reactions, travel and vacation, food care, etc., will be found in Publication No. 567, "Diabetes and You" (revised 1968; 25 cents), from the Superintendent of Documents, U. S. Government Printing Office, Washington, D. C. 20402.

FOREWORD

These recipes are intended to help and guide you in preparing and serving attractive, colorful, unusual, and satisfying meals while conforming to your diabetic diet.

It is important that you follow your doctor's diet orders *explicitly* and use only those recipes suited to your particular suggested caloric intake.

The variety of recipes offered is intended to stimulate your interest in following your diet strictly, as your diet need not be monotonous and unappetizing. Many of these recipes can also be enjoyed by the entire family.

DOCTOR'S PREFACE

Most patients who first learn of having diabetes react with fear, not only to the idea of having a medical disorder, but also to the supposed grim dietary restrictions which they imagine must certainly ensue. To be sure, the more obese patient will require more caloric restriction initially because excess weight is often associated with the need for more stringent maneuvers to obtain precise medical control. Once "ideal weight" is achieved, the cornerstone of good diabetic management is a precise dietary regimen calculated to supply the necessary calories for maintaining this weight.

All too often, new-found diabetics or overweight persons are given a "diet list" of foods allowed, with an admonition to "stay away from sweets." The lack of variety in some of these programs, along with the failure to acquaint the patient with the purpose of diet, brings on a sense of discouragement. Another problem arises with the individual who must eat in restaurants or take a sandwich lunch to work.

This book supplies many helpful bits of dietary information necessary for weight control and diabetic management. The menus are fascinatingly varied, and the general presentation of material should satisfy not only the patient who is able to have his meals prepared at home, but also the individual who is compelled to eat elsewhere. Doctors, too, should find this book a valuable asset in patient education.

Gerson A. Jacobson, M.D.
Torrance, California

AUTHORS' NOTES

We have written this book because many diabetics have expressed their desire for a cookbook with recipes and helpful suggestions specifically related to their dietary needs.

This collection of recipes offers a large variety of unusual and basic recipes which have been kitchen tested and used for hospital patients on diabetic diets. Any of these recipes may be adapted for general use by substituting for the artificial non-caloric sugar substitutes the equivalent amount of regular sugar. Where ingredients which you are unable to tolerate are called for, omit them; the finished product may perhaps be a bit less tasty, but most likely can be eaten with enjoyment just the same.

Each recipe has been carefully calculated to include the caloric content of each measured individual serving, as well as the exchange-group breakdown for each measured individual serving. To help you select recipes suitable for your caloric restrictions, all the recipes have been categorized by calorie count, using asterisks: * 0-100, ** 101-200, *** 201-300 and **** more than 300. The general information chapter includes helpful hints for using diet ingredients, for restaurant dining, and for preparation of box lunches. We have also included reference materials. These include tables of weights and measures, weight tables, diabetic exchange lists, nutritive value of edible parts of food, aids to varying meals, and daily menu guides.

Cookbooks have been published to assist diabetics, but to our knowledge the subject has not been approached from so comprehensive a point of view.

We had you all in mind while writing this, and we hope it will become the most useful book on your cookbook shelf.

Billie Little
Penny Thorup

REMEMBER

that while many people (in addition to your doctor) — a dietitian or nurse for example — can assist you in learning to control diabetes, it is up to YOU to:

1. Continue under medical supervision.

2. Use the exact amount and type of medication prescribed for you! Follow this plan, paying special attention to precise amounts and kinds of foods and the time schedule prescribed for you by your doctor.

3. Use the exact diet plan worked out for you.

4. Do some exercise, in the same amounts, each day.

5. Practice good habits of personal hygiene to minimize the possibility of infection.

EQUIVALENTS BY WEIGHT AND VOLUME

The homemaker who is planning meals for a diabetic needs to know something about food values. The following tables will help determine measurements for carbohydrates, fats, and proteins. Also included are equivalents for most of the measures used in these tables. Be sure to use standard measuring utensils such as an 8-ounce measuring cup, tablespoon, teaspoon, and the like. (The "dime" stores also carry a set of spoons as small as 1/8 of a teaspoon.) It is also a good idea to re-measure *after* cooking. There are a few foods that need not be measured; these will be found in the Exchange Lists.

1 pound (16 ounces)	453.6 grams
1 pound butter or margarine	16 ounces
	4 sticks
	2 cups
	64 pats or squares
1 stick butter or margarine	1/2 cup (approximately)
	16 pats or squares
1000 grams	1 kilogram
1 kilogram	2.2 pounds
1 ounce (fluid or solid)	2 tablespoons
	28.35 grams
1 cup	16 tablespoons
2 cups	1 pint
4 cups	1 quart
4 quarts	1 gallon
16 tablespoons	1 cup
12 tablespoons	3/4 cup
10 tablespoons + 2 teaspoons	2/3 cup
8 tablespoons	1/2 cup
5 tablespoons + 1 teaspoon	1/3 cup
4 tablespoons	1/4 cup
2 tablespoons	1/8 cup
	1 fluid ounce
	28.35 grams
1 tablespoon	3 teaspoons
	14.28 grams
3 teaspoons	1 tablespoon
Dash, or "few grains"	Up to 1/8 teaspoon

CALORIES

1 gram carbohydrate .... 4 calories
1 gram fat... 9 calories
1 gram protein .... 4 calories
1 cup non-dairy whips ....160 (approximately)

GENERAL RULES

MEASURING FOOD:
All food should be measured. You will need a standard 8-ounce measuring cup and a measuring teaspoon and tablespoon. All measurements are level. Most foods are measured after cooking.

FOOD PREPARATION:
Meats may be baked, boiled, broiled or roasted. Do not fry foods except in fat exchange allowed for that meal. Vegetables may be prepared with the family meals, but the portion for the diabetic should be removed before extra fat exchanges or bread exchanges are added.

SPECIAL FOODS:
It is not necessary to buy special foods. Select the diet from the same foods purchased for the rest of the family — milk, vegetables, bread, meats, fats, and fruit (fresh, dried, or canned without sugar). "Special dietetic foods" should be used with discretion; be sure to read labels carefully to determine ingredients. Additional calories in special diet foods must also be figured in the diet.

EXCHANGE LISTS

Special Note:
In figuring the exchanges for the recipes
in this book, exchanges less than 1/8
have been disregarded.

Your doctor will select items from these food groups according to their carbohydrate, fat, and protein content, calorie count, etc. To insure good nutrition, your diet should include the same essential food, sometimes referred to as the "basic four," recommended for everyone.

Breads and Cereals: Whole-grain, enriched, or restored
Fruits and Vegetables
Meat
Milk

The foods on each list have about the same nutritional value. The groupings are called "exchange lists" because one food may be exchanged for another on the same list, BUT food on one list may NOT be exchanged for foods on another list. Each diet plan includes foods from all exchange lists to give variety.

LIST 1 (allowed as desired)
(need not be measured)

Seasonings: Cinnamon, celery salt, garlic, garlic salt, lemon, mustard, mint, nutmeg, parsley, pepper, saccharin and other sugarless sweeteners, spices, vanilla, and vinegar.

Other Foods: Coffee or tea (without sugar or cream), fat-free broth, bouillon, unflavored gelatin, rennet tablets, sour or dill pickles, cranberries (without sugar), rhubarb (without sugar).

Vegetables: Group A — insignificant carbohydrate or calories. Eat as much as desired of raw vegetable; if cooked, limit amount to 1 cup.

Asparagus	Lettuce
Broccoli	Mushrooms
Brussels sprouts	Okra
Cabbage	Peppers, green or red
Cauliflower	Radishes
Celery	Sauerkraut
Chicory	Squash, summer
Cucumbers	String beans
Eggplant	Tomatoes
Escarole	Watercress
Greens: beet, chard, collard, dandelion, kale, mustard, spinach, turnip	

LIST 2 Vegetable Exchanges
Each portion supplies approximately 7 gm of carbohydrate and 2 gm of protein, or 36 calories.

Vegetables: Group B — One serving equals 1/2 cup or 100 gm

Beets	Pumpkin
Carrots	Rutabagas
Onions	Squash, winter
Peas, green	Turnips

LIST 3 Fruit Exchanges
(fresh, dried, or canned without sugar)

Each portion supplies approximately 10 gm of carbohydrate, or 40 calories.

	Household Measurement	Weight of portion
Apple	1 small (2" dia.)	80 gm
Applesauce	1/2 cup	100 gm
Apricots, fresh	2 med.	100 gm
Apricots, dried	4 halves	20 gm
Banana	1/2 small	50 gm
Berries	1 cup	150 gm
Blueberries	2/3 cup	100 gm
Cantaloupe	1/4 (6" dia.)	200 gm
Cherries	10 large	75 gm
Dates	2	15 gm
Figs, fresh	2 large	50 gm
Figs, dried	1 small	15 gm
Grapefruit	1/2 small	125 gm
Grapefruit juice	1/2 cup	100 gm
Grapes	12	75 gm
Grape juice	1/4 cup	60 gm
Honeydew melon	1/8 (7")	150 gm
Mango	1/2 small	70 gm
Orange	1 small	100 gm
Orange juice	1/2 cup	100 gm
Papaya	1/3 med.	100 gm
Peach	1 med.	100 gm
Pear	1 small	100 gm
Pineapple	1/2 cup	80 gm
Pineapple juice	1/3 cup	80 gm
Plums	2 med.	100 gm
Prunes, dried	2	25 gm
Raisins	2 tablespoons	15 gm
Tangerine	1 large	100 gm
Watermelon	1 cup	175 gm

LIST 4 Bread Exchanges
Each portion supplies approximately 15 gm of carbohydrate and 2 gm of protein, or 68 calories.

	Household Measurement	Weight of portion
Bread	1 slice	25 gm
Biscuit, roll	1 (2" diameter)	35 gm
Muffin	1 (2" diameter)	35 gm
Cornbread	1 1/2" cube	35 gm
Flour	2 1/2 tablespoons	20 gm
Cereal, cooked	1/2 cup	100 gm
Cereal, dry (flakes or puffed)	3/4 cup	20 gm
Rice or grits, cooked	1/2 cup	100 gm
Spaghetti, noodles, etc.	1/2 cup	100 gm
Crackers, graham	2	20 gm
Crackers, oyster	20 (1/2 cup)	20 gm
Crackers, saltine	5	20 gm
Crackers, soda	3	20 gm
Crackers, round	6-8	20 gm
Vegetables		
Beans (lima, navy, etc.), dry, cooked	1/2 cup	90 gm
Peas (split peas, etc.), dry, cooked	1/2 cup	90 gm
Baked beans, no pork	1/4 cup	50 gm
Corn	1/3 cup	80 gm
Parsnips	2/3 cup	125 gm
Potato, white, baked or boiled	1 (2" diam.)	100 gm
Potatoes, white, mashed	1/2 cup	100 gm
Potatoes, sweet, or yams	1/4 cup	50 gm
Sponge cake, plain	1 1/2" cube	25 gm
Ice cream (Unless specially prepared for diabetics, omit 2 fat exchanges)	1/2 cup	70 gm

LIST 5 Meat Exchanges
Each portion supplies approximately 7 gm of protein and 5 gm of fat, or 73 calories. (30 gm equal 1 ounce)

	Household Measurement	Weight of portion
Meat and poultry (beef, lamb, pork, liver, chicken, etc.) (med. fat)	1 slice (3" x 2" x 1/8")	30 gm
Cold cuts	1 slice (4 1/2" sq., 1/8" thick)	45 gm
Frankfurter	1 (8-9 per lb.)	50 gm
Codfish, mackerel, etc.	1 slice (2" x 2" x 1")	30 gm
Salmon, tuna, crab	1/4 cup	30 gm
Oysters, shrimp, clams	5 small	45 gm
Sardines	3 medium	30 gm
Cheese, cheddar, American	1 slice (3 1/2" x 1 1/2" x 1/4")	30 gm
Cheese, cottage	1/4 cup	45 gm
Egg	1	50 gm
Peanut butter	2 tablespoons	30 gm

Limit peanut butter to one exchange per day unless diet plan allows for carbohydrate.

LIST 6 Fat Exchanges
Each portion supplies approximately 5 gm of fat, or 45 calories.

	Household Measurement	Weight of portion
Butter or margarine	1 tsp.	5 gm
Bacon, crisp	1 slice	10 gm
Cream, light	2 tbsp.	30 gm
Cream, heavy	1 tbsp.	15 gm
Cream cheese	1 tbsp.	15 gm
French dressing	1 tbsp.	15 gm
Mayonnaise	1 tsp.	5 gm
Oil or cooking fat	1 tsp.	5 gm
Nuts	6 small	10 gm
Olives	5 small	50 gm
Avocado	1/8 (4" diam.)	25 gm

LIST 7 Milk Exchanges
Each portion supplies approximately 12 gm of carbohydrate, 8 gm of protein, and 10 gm of fat, or 170 calories.

	Household Measurement	Weight of portion
Milk, whole	1 cup	240 gm
Milk, evaporated	1/2 cup	120 gm
*Milk, powdered	1/4 cup	35 gm
*Buttermilk	1 cup	240 gm
*Milk, skim	1 cup	240 gm

*Add 2 fat exchanges if milk is fat-free.

FOODS TO AVOID:

Sugar
Candy
Honey
Jam
Jelly
Marmalade
Syrups
Fried, scalloped, or creamed foods

Beer, wine, or other alcoholic beverages
Pie
Cake
Cookies
Pastries
Condensed Milk
Soft Drinks
Candy-Coated Gum

EAT ONLY
those foods which are on the diet list.
the amounts of foods on diet.

DO NOT
skip meals.
eat between meals.

The use of the exchange list is based upon the recommendation of the American Dietetic Association and The American Diabetic Association in cooperation with the Diabetes Branch of the U. S. Public Health Service, Department of Health, Education, and Welfare.

NOTES ON SPECIAL INGREDIENTS USED IN RECIPES

1. In order to reduce the caloric content of numerous recipes without affecting quality, we have included various diet ingredients available in local supermarkets. We have calculated the calories and exchange groupings in our recipes using the following diet products:

   diet margarine
   diet mayonnaise
   diet salad dressings
   imitation dairy and non-dairy products
   diet puddings
   diet sauces and toppings

   If you prefer to use an ingredient other than the diet supplement, you will have to adjust the calories and exchanges.

2. **Sweeteners:** No-calorie sweeteners may be substituted for sugar in many recipes, and also used on foods that need a certain amount of sweetening. They are sold in granulated, liquid, and tablet form. Granulated sweetener may be sprinkled on cereals and fresh fruits; it dissolves immediately. For cold beverages the liquid is most convenient, and either the tablet or the granulated may be used in cooking or in hot beverages. For best results, add the sweetening agent toward the end of the cooking process, since the sweetening power is lessened when exposed to high or low temperatures for any long period of time.

   Some sweeteners are available with either a calcium base or a sodium base. Calcium base sweeteners are slightly less sweet than sodium form. They are suggested for the diabetic who is on a low-sodium diet.

   If you find too much substitute has been used, and that it leaves a bitter taste in the mouth, counteract it with a little salt (providing you are permitted salt).

   The many sugar substitutes on the market include Sweeta, Sucaryl, Saccharin, Sweetness and Light, Sweet 'N, Sprinkle Sweet, Sugartwin, Sweet 'n Low, and Ril Sweet. There are others also, which you may prefer.

   For SUBSTITUTE SUGAR SYRUP, combine equal quantities of water and the sugar substitute. Bring to a boil; boil 5 minutes or so. Store in a covered jar in your refrigerator and use for sweetening cold drinks. (This may be used in place of the commercial liquid sweetener.)

Syrups: (May be used to sweeten fruits for canning.)

Light: 7 teaspoons of sugar substitute and 4 cups of water. Boil together 5 minutes. Skim. Makes 4 1/2 cups.

Medium: 13 teaspoons substitute, 3 cups water. Boil 5 minutes. Skim. Makes 3 3/4 cups.

Heavy: 20 teaspoons substitute, 2 cups water. Boil 5 minutes. Skim. Makes 2 2/3 cups.

Glazes: Non-nutritive sweetener equivalent to 1 cup brown sugar; juice and rind (grated) of 1 orange.

Non-nutritive sweetener equivalent to 1 cup sugar; 1/2 cup cider, dietetic maraschino cherry juice or sweet pickle juice.

1 glass dietetic currant jelly, melted.

1/2 cup dietetic orange marmalade, softened.

There are several brown sugar substitutes available, but if you cannot locate any and brown sugar is called for in a recipe, put granulated white sugar substitute in a frying pan over VERY LOW HEAT, and stir constantly until caramelized.

Use bulk non-nutritives for cakes, cookies, bread, etc. For drinks use liquid non-nutritive sweeteners.

Using a liquid rather than a granulated sweetener will reduce the number of cups of sugar in a recipe. For example: 1 1/2 cups of granulated regular sugar, or granulated sugar substitute, is the equivalent of one tablespoon of liquid sweetener.

3. All diet margarines contain less than half the calories of regular margarine — 17 per teaspoon (5 gms), 50 per tablespoon (14 gms). Although it is not recommended for frying, it is, with proper care, usable (first melt *SLOWLY* in a frying pan, add food, cover and cook over *LOW* heat). When baking, remember that it has only half the fat content of regular margarines, so in recipes calling for more than two tablespoons of margarine, we suggest the regular soft-form or stick-form margarines.

4. **Wine and Liquor Notes.** The recipes containing alcohol are not for diabetics without the explicit consent of their own doctor. Each recipe containing beer, liqueurs, liquor, or wine is specially marked.

AIDS TO VARYING MEALS

☐ Bake, broil, or roast meats.
Bake, broil, or poach fish.

☐ Add herbs to meats and vegetables. (Use 1/4 teaspoon dry herbs for each 6 servings of fish, meat, or vegetables.)

☐ Try basil, rosemary, garlic salt, dry mustard, or curry powder with beef or lamb; rosemary or savory with chicken, fish, or veal.

☐ Season tomatoes with curry powder, basil, or oregano; turnips with rosemary; cabbage with savory; zucchini or carrots with thyme or nutmeg; cauliflower with dill; spinach with marjoram or nutmeg.

☐ The addition of seasoning salt and lemon pepper to recipes gives an entirely new taste.

☐ To enhance dishes use a variety of condiments: Chervil for soups and eggs (1/2 teaspoon for 4 servings); Beau Monde for eggs, fish, meats, sauces, and stuffing (1/2 teaspoon for 4 servings).
Mei Yen in shrimp soufflé (1 1/2 teaspoons) or 1 tablespoon to either 4 eggs or 3 cups milk.
Bay leaf, celery salt, or marjoram (1 teaspoon to 1 teaspoon salt) for stews.
Green onion seasoning (1 teaspoon to 4-6 pound chicken).
Tarragon (2 teaspoons to 4-6 pound chicken) for stuffing.

☐ Add herbs and spices to liquids and be sure you thoroughly crush any whole spices such as anise seed, basil, bay leaf, oregano, rosemary, thyme, etc., or in the case of leaves, such as bay leaf, remove before serving.

☐ Interesting meals may be prepared if you are careful in selecting from your exchange lists. For instance, you may prepare a stew if you select one small potato from the Bread Exchange (List 4). . .vegetables and meat may be added according to your own meal plan; or you might wish to have a spaghetti dinner by using spaghetti from Bread Exchange (List 1) or (List 2), cheese from Meat Exchange (List 5) and meat sauce.

☐ Soy margarine or Soyamaise are good substitutes for margarine or butter as there is less fat content (if you are able to tolerate soy derivatives).

☐ Use nondairy whips. Each cup averages about 160 calories.

☐ Good sauces may be made from Sweet 'n Sour Barbecue Sauce or Teriyaki Barbecue Marinade, but be sure to check the sugar content.

☐ Low-calorie diet spreads are available and may be used for sandwiches, hors d'oeuvres, etc.

☐ Unusual low-calorie or water-packed fruits such as bing cherries, fruits for salads, Kadota figs, mandarin oranges, pineapple spears, purple plums, etc., are also available.

ADDITIONAL SUGGESTIONS

☐ Measure dry ingredients before liquid; this will save washing utensils!

☐ Sift flour **before** you measure when the recipe calls for sifted flour. Sift the flour into a bowl, then spoon into measuring utensil. Level with a spatula or knife.

☐ Molasses or syrup flow more easily if measuring utensil is rinsed in cold water and then lightly greased.

☐ 1 medium egg = 1/4 cup eggs.

☐ Have eggs at room temperature.

☐ Arrowroot: 1 tablespoon = 1 slice of bread. (May be used for fruit juices.)

☐ Arrowroot powder may be used in place of flour. In recipes where we use arrowroot, flour may also be used, but be sure to double the amount.

☐ Cornstarch: 2 tablespoons = 1 slice bread. (May be used for fruit juices.)

☐ Egg Yolk: Use this in place of 1 tablespoon flour. (Yields 3 gms protein and 5 gms fat, no carbohydrate.)

☐ Flour: 1 tablespoon = 1/3 slice of bread. (Use all-purpose flour, sifted.) 2 1/2 tablespoons = 1 slice bread. (Use all-purpose flour, sifted.)

☐ Tapioca: 1 teaspoon, no exchange necessary. (This is used mostly for sweet sauces. In thickening power this is equivalent to 1 tablespoon flour.)

EATING OUT

Suggestions for restaurant dining and for preparing lunches to be eaten away from home

The questions frequently asked by people on diabetic diets is, "How do I make this diet fit my normal, daily routine?" This is extremely important both to children and adults. Size of portions will depend upon individual calorie requirements and allowed food exchanges.

LUNCH-BOX MEALS

1. Bread exchange: use either bread or crackers.
2. Fat exchange: butter or mayonnaise; cream for beverages.
3. Fruit exchange: use fresh fruit, unsweetened canned fruits, or fruit juices.
4. Meat exchange: hard-boiled eggs, cold cuts, roast beef, turkey, chicken, ham, cheese, cottage cheese, peanut butter.
5. Milk exchange: as beverage.
6. Vegetables List 1 or 2: raw vegetables such as carrots, celery, cherry tomatoes, cucumber sticks, green pepper rings, radishes, whole tomatoes.

LUNCH-BOX SUGGESTIONS

Sandwich: composed of bread exchange (1 or 2 slices of bread), meat exchange (turkey or beef), fat exchange (butter or mayonnaise), and lettuce, sliced tomato, or other vegetable.

Sandwich fillings: for people on high-calorie diets, use chicken, egg, or tuna salad, for example.

Snacks: graham crackers and butter
cheese and crackers
peanut butter and crackers
crackers and cold cuts, fish, or poultry.

EXAMPLES

Milk (thermos or purchased at school)

Sandwich of turkey, peanut butter, etc.

Fresh fruit, apple or tangerine

Carrot and celery sticks

Sandwich or cheese and crackers or cottage cheese

Fresh fruit, pear

Fresh tomato

Coffee with cream, or milk

HOT LUNCH PROGRAMS

Straight meat entrees with vegetables

or

Plain hamburger sandwich

or

Plain hot dog on a bun

Fresh fruit

Salad without salad dressing

Beverages, fruit juice or milk, coffee or tea

Assorted List 1: raw vegetable relishes

Cold baked chicken

Bread and butter

Fresh fruit

Milk or hot beverage, as desired

DINING OUT HINTS

It can be easy to dine out on your calorie-restricted diet comfortably if you keep your exchange groupings in mind. Avoid dishes you are unsure of, such as casseroles, creamed foods, and other dishes that might have "hidden" ingredients.

1. Order plain soups such as consommés, French onion, vegetable.

2. When ordering a salad, ask for your dressing to be brought in a side dish so you can measure the amount according to the fat exchanges you are allowed for that meal. If your fat exchanges are limited, lemon wedges or vinegar (wine or cider) are usually available upon request.
   Sliced tomatoes are usually available upon request. Order them without dressing or with the dressing in a side dish.

3. In selecting entrees, take meat items that are either baked, broiled, poached, or roasted. Ask the restaurant to eliminate butter from their preparation. The following are recommended:
   a. Baked or broiled chicken.
   b. Broiled shish kabob or brochette without marinade.
   c. Broiled or baked seafood or fish.
   d. Broiled steak.
   e. Hamburger steak.
   f. Prime rib, roast beef.
   g. Roast turkey (omit dressing and gravy).

Request that sauces and gravies be eliminated from your entree or brought separately.

4. Order hot and cold cereals plain. Use milk or cream on cereals according to your exchange pattern.

5. Order bread or rolls without fat, according to exchange pattern. Order toast dry.

6. Plain potatoes are readily available either baked or boiled. For oven browned or mashed potato, figure one bread exchange plus one fat exchange.

7. Order cooked vegetables plain; if not available figure one extra fat exchange per serving of vegetables.

8. Recommended vegetables commonly served in restaurants include green beans, tomatoes, carrots, peas, corn on the cob, mixed vegetables, asparagus.

9. Broiled steak is often suitable for breakfast.

10. Order eggs poached or soft cooked; for fried or scrambled eggs, if prepared in a skillet, add one fat exchange.

11. Order bacon or sausage crisp.

12. Fresh fruit is usually available (in season); choose banana, half grapefruit (plain), melon wedge, or fresh strawberries. Stewed prunes are often available without sugar syrup.

13. Order unsweetened fruit juice, or fresh fruit juice.

EXAMPLES

Breakfast

1/2 fresh grapefruit
3/4 cup cold cereal with cream or milk
1 poached egg

1 slice dry toast
1 strip crisp bacon
1 pat butter
Coffee or tea

OR

1/2 glass fresh orange juice
1/2 cup oatmeal with cream or milk
1 fried egg prepared in pan with 1 pat butter

1 strip bacon
Dry toast
Butter
Coffee or tea

Lunch

Tossed green salad with French
dressing or wine vinegar
Broiled hamburger steak
Toasted dry bun

Sliced tomatoes
Cantaloupe wedge
Milk, coffee, tea

OR

Cup of bouillon or French onion
soup

Chef's salad with dressing in side
dish

OR

Crab Louis with dressing in side
dish
Dinner roll or soda cracker

Butter
Fruit juice or serving of fresh
fruit

Dinner

Green or spinach salad, or salad
of your choice without dress-
ing
Dressing of your choice in side
dish
Broiled New York Steak or
Prime Rib au jus
Baked potato
Green beans
Dinner roll or bread
Milk or hot beverage
Fruit as desired, or later at home.

OR

Tomato or "V-8" juice cocktail
Fresh fruit cup or melon wedge
Broiled lobster tail, butter in side
dish
Mashed potatoes or potato
Broiled tomato
Dinner roll or crackers
Milk or beverage

OR

Tossed salad with dressing separate
Charcoal broiled hamburger
sandwich, plain (have condiments brought separately)
Milk or beverage
Fruit as desired, or later at home

DAILY MENU GUIDE

The sample diets listed below show some of the ways that the exchange lists may be used to add variety to your meals. Use the exchange lists to plan different menus.

CALORIE DIETS

The following suggested diets include a breakdown of exchange lists for breakfast, lunch, and dinner. Liquid diets are suggested to replace any meal for those who are sick or dieting.

1000 CALORIES (approximately)	carbohydrate	90 gm
	protein	60 gm
	fat	45 gm

LIQUID DIET

Full Liquid:
```
Eggnog(milk.................1/2 cup ...............120 gm
       (egg .................1 .......................  50 gm
Orange juice .................3/4 cup ...............150 gm
Milk .........................3/4 cup ...............180 gm
```

Clear Liquid:
```
Clear bouillon.................1 cup
Orange juice .................1 cup ...............200 gm
Gelatin dessert .............1/2 cup ...............100 gm
```

Bedtime Feeding (when directed by doctor):

1/2 milk exchange (1/2 cup milk)

1/2 bread exchange (2 crackers)

will add approximately 120 calories to the daily diet.

BREAKFAST

1 fruit exchange (List 3)
1 bread exchange (List 4)
1 meat exchange (List 5)
1 milk exchange (List 7)
Coffee or tea (any amount)

Example:
```
Orange juice .................1/2 cup
Toast ...........................1 slice
Egg..............................1
Milk, whole..................1 cup
```

18

LUNCH

2 meat exchanges (List 5)
1 1/2 bread exchanges (List 4)
Vegetable(s) as desired (List 1)
1 fruit exchange (List 3)
1 milk (skim) exchange
  (List 7)
2 fat exchanges (List 6)
Coffee or tea (any amount)

Example:

Meat...........................2 slices
  (3" x 2" x 1/8" ea.)
Potatoes ....1/2 cup
Lettuce and tomato
  salad ....as desired
Bread...........................1/2 slice
Pineapple...................1/2 cup
Milk, skim ....1 cup
French dressing............1 tbsp.

DINNER

2 meat exchanges (List 5)
1 1/2 bread exchanges (List 4)
Vegetable(s) as desired (List 1)
1 vegetable exchange (List 2)
1 fruit exchange (List 3)
1 fat exchange (List 6)
Coffee or tea (any amount)

Example:

Tomato juice ....3 oz.
Chicken......................2 slices
  (3" x 2" x 1/8" ea.)
Noodles.......................1/2 cup
Asparagus....................as desired
Peas...........................1/2 cup
Bread...........................1/2 slice
Butter ....1/2 tsp.
Banana......................1/2 small

1200 CALORIES (approximately)

carbohydrate	125 gm
protein	60 gm
fat	50 gm

LIQUID DIET

Full Liquid:

Eggnog(milk...................1/2 cup ....120 gm
  (egg ....1 .... 50 gm
Orange juice..................1 cup ....200 gm
Milk ....3/4 cup ....180 gm

Clear Liquid:

Clear bouillon.................1 cup
Orange juice 1   cup ....200 gm
Grapefruit juice..............1/2 cup ....100 gm
Gelatin dessert ....1/2 cup ....100 gm

Bedtime Feeding (when directed by physician):

1/2 milk exchange (1/2 cup
  milk)

1/2 bread exchange (2 crackers)

} will add approximately 120 calories to the daily diet.

BREAKFAST
1 fruit exchange (List 3)
1 bread exchange (List 4)
2 meat exchanges (List 5)
1/2 milk exchange (List 7)

Example:
Orange juice ....1/2 cup
Toast ....1 slice
Eggs 2
Milk, whole.................1/2 cup

LUNCH
2 meat exchanges (List 5)
1 bread exchange (List 4)
Vegetable(s) as desired
    (List 1)
1 fruit exchange (List 3)
1/2 milk (skim)
    exchange (List 7)
1 fat exchange (List 6)
Coffee or tea (any amount)

Example:
Meat..........................2 slices
    (3" x 2" x 1/8" ea.)
Broccoli.......................as desired
Lettuce and tomato
    salad.......................as desired
Bread..........................1 slice
Butter ....1 tsp.
Pineapple.....................1/2 cup
Milk, skim ....1/2 cup

DINNER
2 meat exchanges (List 5)
1 bread exchange (List 4)
Vegetable(s) as desired (List 1)
1 vegetable exchange (List 2)
1 fruit exchange (List 3)
1 fat exchange (List 6)
Coffee or tea (any amount)

Example:
Tomato juice ....3 oz.
Chicken.....................2 slices
    (3" x 2" x 1/8" ea.)
Noodles.......................1/2 cup
Asparagus....................as desired
Peas...........................1/2 cup
Butter ....1 tsp.
Banana......................1/2 small

1500 CALORIES (approximately)	carbohydrate	150 gm
	protein	70 gm
	fat	70 gm

LIQUID DIET

Full Liquid:
Eggnog(milk.................1/2 cup ....120 gm
    (egg.....................1 .... 50 gm
Orange juice ....1 cup ....200 gm
Gelatin dessert ....1/2 cup ....100 gm
Milk ....1/2 cup ....120 gm

Clear Liquid:
```
Bouillon (if desired) .........1 cup
Orange juice ..................1 cup ...................200 gm
Grapefruit juice..............1/2 cup ...................100 gm
    with sugar.................2 tsp. ...................... 10 gm
Gelatin dessert ...............1/2 cup ...................100 gm
```

Bedtime Feeding (when directed by physician):

1/2 milk exchange (1/2 cup milk)

1/2 bread exchange (2 crackers)

} will add approximately 120 calories to the daily diet.

BREAKFAST
2 fruit exchanges (List 3)
2 bread exchanges (List 4)
2 meat exchanges (List 5)
1 milk exchange (List 7)
2 fat exchanges (List 6)
Coffee or tea (any amount)

Example:
```
Orange juice ................1 cup
Toast ..........................2 slices
Eggs ...........................2
Bacon, crisp ................1 slice
Milk ...........................1 cup
Butter .........................1 tsp.
```

LUNCH
2 meat exchanges (List 5)
2 bread exchanges (List 4)
Vegetable(s) as desired (List 1)
1 vegetable exchange (List 2)
1 fruit exchange (List 3)
1 milk exchange (List 7)
1 fat exchange (List 6)
Coffee or tea (any amount)

Example:
```
Cold cuts.....................1 slice
   (4 1/2" sq. x 1/8" thick)
Bread...........................2 slices
Butter .........................1 tsp.
Lettuce salad with
   cottage cheese...........1/4 cup
Beets...........................1/2 cup
Pear............................1 small
Milk ...........................1 cup
```

DINNER
2 meat exchanges (List 5)
2 bread exchanges (List 4)
Vegetable(s) as desired (List 1)
1 vegetable exchange (List 2)
1 fruit exchange (List 3)
1 milk exchange (List 7)
1 fat exchange (List 6)
Coffee or tea (any amount)

Example:
```
Roast Beef ...................2 slices
   (3" x 2" x 1/8" ea.)
Potatoes .....................1/2 cup
Squash .......................1/2 cup
Relish--celery,
   radishes .................as desired
Bread..........................1 slice
Butter .........................1 tsp.
Cherries......................10 large
Milk ...........................1 cup
```

1800 CALORIES (approximately)   carbohydrate   180 gm
                                      protein   80 gm
                                      fat   80 gm

LIQUID DIET

Full Liquid:
    Eggnog (milk.................2/3 cup ....160 gm
            (egg ....1 .... 50 gm
    Orange juice ....1 cup ....200 gm
    Custard (milk ....1/2 cup ....120 gm
            (egg ....1 .... 50 gm
    Grape juice ....3/4 cup ....180 gm

Clear Liquid:
    Orange juice ....1 cup ....200 gm
        with sugar..................2 tsp. .... 10 gm
    Grapefruit juice...............1/2 cup ....100 gm
        with sugar.................2 tsp. .... 10 gm
    Gelatin dessert ....1/2 cup ....100 gm

Bedtime Feeding (when directed by physician):
    1/2 milk exchange (1/2 cup
      milk)   will add approximately 120
                                     calories to the daily diet.
    1/2 bread exchange (2 crack-
    ers)

BREAKFAST	Example:
2 fruit exchanges (List 3)	Orange juice ....1 cup
2 bread exchanges (List 4)	Toast ....2 slices
2 meat exchanges (List 5)	Eggs 2
1 milk exchange (List 7)	Bacon, crisp ....1 slice
2 fat exchanges (List 6)	Milk ....1 cup
Coffee or tea (any amount)	Butter ....1 tsp.

LUNCH	Example:
2 meat exchanges (List 5)	Cold cuts......................1 slice
2 bread exchanges (List 4)	(4 1/2" sq. x 1/8" thick)
Vegetable(s) as desired (List 1)	Bread ....2 slices
1 vegetable exchange (List 2)	Butter ....1 tsp.
1 fruit exchange (List 3)	Lettuce salad with
1 milk exchange (List 7)	cottage cheese ....1/4 cup
1 fat exchange (List 6)	Beets...........................1/2 cup
Coffee or tea (any amount)	Pear...........................1 small
	Milk ....1 cup

DINNER

2 meat exchanges (List 5)
2 bread exchanges (List 4)
Vegetable(s) as desired (List 1)
1 vegetable exchange (List 2)
1 fruit exchange (List 3)
1 milk exchange (List 7)
1 fat exchange (List 6)
Coffee or tea (any amount)

Example:

Roast Beef ....2 slices
   (3" x 2" x 1/8" ea.)
Potatoes ....1/2 cup
Squash ....1/2 cup
Relish--celery,
   radishes...................as desired
Bread ....1 slice
Butter ....1 tsp.
Cherries......................10 large
Milk ....1 cup

2000 CALORIES (approximately)

carbohydrate	210 gm
protein	90 gm
fat	90 gm

LIQUID DIET

Full Liquid:

Milk   (milk ....1/2 cup ....120 gm
Toast (bread ....1 slice......................... 25 gm
Eggnog(milk...................1/2 cup ....120 gm
    (egg ....1 .... 50 gm
Milk ....1 cup ....240 gm
Orange juice ....1 cup ....200 gm

Clear Liquid:

Orange juice ....1 cup ....200 gm
   with sugar...................2 tsp. .... 10 gm
Grapefruit juice...................1 cup ....200 gm
   with sugar...................2 tsp. .... 10 gm
Gelatin dessert ....1/2 cup ....100 gm

Bedtime Feeding (when directed by physician):

1/2 milk exchange (1/2 cup milk)
1/2 bread exchange (2 crackers)
} will add approximately 120 calories to the daily diet.

BREAKFAST

1 fruit exchange (List 3)
3 bread exchanges (List 4)
2 meat exchanges (List 5)
1 milk exchange (List 7)
2 fat exchanges (List 6)
Coffee or tea (any amount)

Example:

Orange 1
Cereal, cooked..............1 cup
Toast ....1 slice
Eggs 2
Butter ....1 tsp.
Bacon, crisp ....1 slice
Milk ....1 cup

LUNCH

2 meat exchanges (List 5)
2 bread exchanges (List 4)
Vegetable(s) as desired (List 1)
1 vegetable exchange (List 2)
2 fruit exchanges (List 3)
1 milk exchange (List 7)
2 fat exchanges (List 6)
Coffee or tea (any amount)

Example:

Cold cuts......................2 slices
  (4 1/2" sq. x 1/8" thick)
Baked potato.................1 (2")
Asparagus....................as desired
Carrots........................1/2 cup
Bread...........................1 slice
Butter ....2 tsp.
Apricots ....1 cup
Milk ....1 cup

DINNER

3 meat exchanges (List 5)
2 bread exchanges (List 4)
Vegetable(s) as desired (List 1)
1 vegetable exchange (List 2)
2 fruit exchanges (List 3)
1 milk exchange (List 7)
2 fat exchanges (List 6)
Coffee or tea (any amount)

Example:

Liver, broiled................3 slices
  (3" x 2" x 1/8" ea.)
Potatoes ....1/2 cup
Onions ....1/2 cup
Broccoli.......................as desired
Bread...........................1 slice
Butter ....1 tsp.
Banana........................1 small
  with cream...............1 oz.
Milk ....1 cup

2200 CALORIES (approximately)

carbohydrate 250 Gm.
protein 90 Gm.
fat 90 Gm.

LIQUID DIET

Full Liquid:

Milk   (milk......................1/2 cup ....120 gm
Toast (bread ....1 1/2 slices........................ 38 gm
Eggnog or (milk ....1/2 cup ....120 gm
Custard (egg ....1.. 50 gm
Milk ....1 cup ....240 gm
Orange juice ....1 cup ....200 gm
  with sugar.....................2 tsp................................... 10 gm

Clear Liquid:

Orange juice ....1 cup ....200 gm
  with sugar.....................2 tsp................................... 10 gm
Grapefruit juice...................1 cup ....200 gm
  with sugar.....................2 tsp................................... 10 gm
Orange juice ....1/2 cup ....100 gm
Gelatin dessert ....1/3 cup .... 65 gm

Bedtime Feeding (when directed by physician):

1/2 milk exchange (1/2 cup milk) ⎫

1/2 bread exchange (2 crackers) ⎬ will add approximately 120 calories to the daily diet.

BREAKFAST
2 fruit exchanges (List 3)
3 1/2 bread exchanges (List 4)
2 meat exchanges (List 5)
1 milk exchange (List 7)
2 fat exchanges (List 6)
Coffee or tea (any amount)

Example:
Orange juice ....1 cup
Cornflakes ....3/4 cup
Toast ....2 1/2 slices
Eggs 2
Butter ....1 tsp.
Cream.........................1 oz.
Milk ....1 cup

LUNCH
2 meat exchanges (List 5)
4 bread exchanges (List 4)
Vegetable(s) as desired (List 1)
1 fruit exchange (List 3)
1 milk exchange (List 7)
2 fat exchanges (List 6)
Coffee or tea (any amount)

Example:
Cheese.................1 oz.
Bread...............2 slices, sandwich
Butter .... 1 tsp.
Roast Beef .... 1 slice
      (3" x 2" x 1/8")
Bread...............2 slices, sandwich
Mayonnaise......... 1 tsp.
Celery and radishes........as desired
Apple...........................1 small
Milk ....1 cup

DINNER
2 meat exchanges (List 5)
3 bread exchanges (List 4)
Vegetable(s) as desired (List 1)
1 vegetable exchange (List 2)
2 fruit exchanges (List 3)
1 milk exchange (List 7)
2 fat exchanges (List 6)
Coffee or tea (any amount)

Example:
Hamburger...................2 patties
      (3" diam., 1/4" thick ea.)
Whole-kernel corn ....1/3 cup
Tomatoes....................as desired
Carrots.......................1/2 cup
Bread ....2 slices
Butter ....2 tsp.
Plums.........................4 med.
Milk ....1 cup

2500 CALORIES (approximately)   carbohydrate   250 gm
                                     protein   100 gm
                                     fat   120 gm

Bedtime Feeding (when directed by physician):

1/2 milk exchange (1/2 cup milk)
1/2 bread exchange (2 crackers)

will add approximately 120 calories to the daily diet.

BREAKFAST
2 fruit exchanges (List 3)
3 1/2 bread exchanges (List 4)
3 meat exchanges (List 5)
1 milk exchange (List 7)
3 fat exchanges (List 6)
Coffee or tea (any amount)

Example:
Orange juice ....1 cup
Cereal, cooked ....3/4 cup
Toast ....2 slices
Eggs 2
Ham ....1 slice
    (3" x 2" x 1/8")
Butter ....2 tsp.
Cream ....1 oz.
Milk ....1 cup

DINNER
2 meat exchanges (List 5)
3 bread exchanges (List 4)
Vegetable(s) as desired (List 1)
1 vegetable exchange (List 2)
2 fruit exchanges (List 3)
1 milk exchange (List 7)
4 fat exchanges (List 6)
Coffee or tea (any amount)

Example:
Grapefruit juice.............1 cup
Tuna fish ....1/2 cup
   with mayonnaise........2 tsp.
Potato, baked ....1 (2")
   with butter ....1 tsp.
Peas...........................1/2 cup
Lettuce salad ....as desired
Bread.........................2 slices
Butter ....1 tsp.
Pear...........................1 small
Milk ....1 cup

3000 CALORIES (approximately)   carbohydrate   300 gm
                                       protein   130 gm
                                     fat   140 gm

BREAKFAST
2 fruit exchanges (List 3)
2 bread exchanges (List 4)
2 meat exchanges (List 5)
1 milk exchange (List 7)

Example:
Orange juice ....1 cup
Cereal, cooked ....1/2 cup
Toast ....1 slice
Egg.............................1

3 fat exchanges (List 6)
Coffee or tea (any amount)

Ham ....1 slice
   (3" x 2" x 1/8")
Butter ....2 tsp.
Milk ....1 cup
Cream, light ....2 tbsp.

LUNCH
3 meat exchanges (List 5)
4 bread exchanges (List 4)
Vegetable(s) as desired (List 1)
2 fruit exchanges (List 3)
1 milk exchange (List 7)
2 fat exchanges (List 6)
Coffee or tea (any amount)

Example:
Egg, hard-cooked and
   chopped...................1
   mixed with
   mayonnaise ....1 tsp.
Bread ....2 slices
Luncheon meat ....2 slices
   (4 1/2" sq. x 1/8" thick ea.)
Mayonnaise..................1 tsp.
Bread ....2 slices
Dill pickle, sliced;
   radishes ....as desired
Orange 1
Milk ....1 cup
Apple...........................1 small

MIDAFTERNOON FEEDING
1 meat exchange (List 5)
1 bread exchange (List 4)
1/2 milk exchange (List 7)
1 fat exchange (List 6)

Example:
American cheese............1 slice
   (3 1/2" x 1 1/2" x 1/4")
Soda crackers 3
Butter ....1 tsp.
Milk ....1/2 cup
Coffee or tea ....(any
               amount)

DINNER
3 meat exchanges (List 5)
4 bread exchanges (List 4)
Vegetable(s) as desired (List 1)
1 vegetable exchange (List 2)
2 fruit exchanges (List 3)
1 milk exchange (List 7)
3 fat exchanges (List 6)
Coffee or tea (any amount)

Example:
Grapefruit juice.............1/2 cup
Tuna fish ....3/4 cup
Potato, baked ....1 (4")
   with butter ....1 tsp.
Peas...........................1/2 cup
Lettuce salad ....as desired
Bread ....2 slices
Butter ....2 tsp.
Pear............................1 small
Milk ....1 cup

BEDTIME FEEDING
2 bread exchanges (List 4)
2 meat exchanges (List 5)
1 fat exchange (List 6)

Example:
Rye bread ....2 slices
Ham ....2 slices
   (3" x 2" x 1/8" ea.)
Mayonnaise..................1 tsp.

APPETIZERS AND BEVERAGES

* - 0 - 100 Calories
** - 101 - 200 Calories
*** - 201 - 300 Calories
**** - More than 301 Calories

100 grams are equivalent to 3 1/2 ounces. This makes one serving when prepared according to the directions on the label.

When using basic ingredients such as arrowroot, eggs, flour, margarine, and tapioca, refer to General Information and to Table of Weights and Measures.

*APPLE FOAM

Exchanges per serving: 1 cup = 1/2 fruit.
Calories per serving: 20   Yield: 2 servings

2 cups apple juice
1 teaspoon lemon juice
1/4 cup (1-2 medium) egg whites

Non-nutritive sweetener equivalent to 1 1/2 cups sugar
1/16 teaspoon cinnamon

Chill juices. Beat egg whites until stiff; add sweetener while beating. Add apple and lemon juices; pour into fruit cups. Mix sugar substitute and cinnamon, enough to sprinkle on fruit juice mixture.

*HONOLULU DIP

Exchanges per serving: 1/4 cup = 1/2 fat, 1/4 fruit.
Calories per serving: 43 (for dip only)   Yield: 1 1/3 cups

1/2 cup chopped fresh (or crushed, artificially sweetened) pineapple
2 tablespoons chopped mint

3 ounces cream cheese
2 tablespoons safflower mayonnaise

Blend ingredients together and serve with crisp carrot and celery sticks and crackers.

*CHEESE NIBBLERS

Exchanges per serving: 1 ball = 1/4 bread, 2/3 fat, 1/4 meat.
Calories per serving: 60   Yield: 36 nibblers

1/2 cup sharp cheddar cheese, grated
1/2 cup diet margarine
1 cup flour

Mix the ingredients together and roll into balls. These can be made ahead of time and frozen — just freeze on a cookie sheet and then store in bags. To bake, place them, frozen, in an oven that has been preheated to 375° for 20-25 minutes.

*GOLDEN SHOYU DIP

Exchanges per serving: 2 tablespoons = 2 fat.
Calories per serving: 90   Yield: 1 1/4 cups

1 cup safflower mayonnaise
1/4 cup soy sauce
1/2 teaspoon instant onion
1/4 teaspoon arrowroot powder

Blend all ingredients until smooth. Chill and restir before serving as dip for all fish "pupus" or with grilled or fried fish.

**RUMAKI

Exchanges per serving: 4 Rumaki = 2 fat, 1/2 meat.
Calories per serving: 120   Yield: 48 Rumakis

12 chicken livers (see note)
1 teaspoon seasoned salt
1/8 teaspoon ginger
1 cup water chestnuts, drained
16 slices bacon

Cut livers into small bite-size pieces and season with salt and ginger; cut water chestnuts into halves and bacon into thirds; wrap a piece of liver and a half chestnut in bacon and secure with a pick. Broil or bake in 425° oven until golden brown (25-30 minutes). Serve hot with fruit chutney, chili sauce, Chinese Mustard, or Hot Shoyu Sauce.

Note: Chicken livers can be eliminated and just the water chestnuts fixed as above, in which case omit meat exchange.

***CHEESE AND PINEAPPLE PUPUS

Exchanges per serving: 1/3 cup dip = 3 fat, 1/2 meat,
                 1/2 cup pineapple = 1 fruit.
Calories per serving: 225   Yield: Fruit, 2 cups
                                        Sauce, 3 cups

1 fresh pineapple, cubed
1 1/2 cups Luau mayonnaise
1 cup cheddar cheese, grated
1/2 cup shredded coconut

Serve pineapple chunks on picks with bowls of other ingredients. Dip pineapple first in mayonnaise, then in cheese and coconut.

*CRANBERRY SIP

Exchanges per serving: 1/2 cup = 3/4 fruit.

Calories per serving: 30   Yield: 2 1/2 cups

1 cup cranberries, washed
1 1/2 cloves, whole
1 teaspoon cinnamon
1 cup water

Non-nutritive sweetener
  equivalent to 1 1/2 cups
  sugar
1/4 cup orange juice
1/4 cup lemon juice
1/16 teaspoon salt

Combine cranberries, spices, water, and sweetener; cook until cranberry skins burst. Strain and add rest of ingredients. Chill.

*LOU'S LEMONADE

Exchanges per serving: 1/2 cup = 1/2 fruit.

Calories per serving: 20   Yield: 8 cups

1 cup unsweetened lemon
  juice
Non-nutritive sweetener
  equivalent to 3/4 cup sugar

6 cups water
1 cup low-calorie cranberry
  juice cocktail

Combine ingredients and mix well. Add ice cubes just prior to serving.

*QUICK DRINK

Exchanges per serving: 1 cup = 1/2 fruit, 1 skim milk.

Calories per serving: 100   Yield: 1 1/4 cups

2/3 cup dry instant powdered
  milk
1/2 cup frozen fruit, unsweetened

Non-nutritive sweetener
  equivalent to 2 tablespoons
  sugar
2 ice cubes

1/8 cup water

Blend in blender until ice cubes are dissolved.

*HOT CHOCOLATE

Exchanges per serving: 1/2 cup = 1/2 fat, 1/2 skim milk.

Calories per serving: 58   Yield: 2 1/2 cups

1 1/2 ounces unsweetened
  chocolate
3/4 cup water
1/16 teaspoon salt

Non-nutritive sweetener
  equivalent to 1/2 cup sugar
2 1/4 cups skim milk

Combine chocolate, water and cook, stirring constantly until chocolate is melted. Add salt and sweetener; bring to boiling point and boil 4 minutes, stirring constantly. Place over boiling water, and gradually add milk, still stirring constantly. Heat. Just before serving beat with rotary beater until frothy.

*APRICOT ORANGE PUNCH

Exchanges per serving: 1/2 cup = 1 fruit.
Calories per serving: 40   Yield: 7 cups

1 1/2 cups unsweetened apricot nectar
3 cups fresh orange juice
1/2 cup fresh lemon juice

Non-nutritive sweetener equivalent to 1/2 cup sugar
2 cups low-calorie ginger ale

Combine first four ingredients. Chill well and just before placing in punch bowl, add well-chilled ginger ale.

*"DELISHUS" PUNCH

Exchanges per serving: 1/2 cup = 1 fruit.
Calories per serving: 40   Yield: 8 cups

1 dozen cloves, whole
1 orange, thinly sliced
1 lemon, thinly sliced
4 cups low-calorie cranberry juice cocktail

1 cinnamon stick
1 teaspoon allspice
2 tablespoons lemon juice
Non-nutritive sweetener to taste

Put a clove in each slice of lemon and orange. Place in a pitcher. Combine cocktail, cinnamon, and allspice and heat to boiling over low heat. Add lemon juice. Add sweetener to taste and strain hot into pitcher over the fruit. Serve in punch cups garnished with fruit slices.

*NONNIE'S CRANBERRY COCKTAIL

Exchanges per serving: 1 cup = 1 fruit.
Calories per serving: 40   Yield: 5 cups

4 cups low-calorie cranberry juice
3 cloves
1 stick cinnamon
1/16 teaspoon salt

Non-nutritive sweetener equivalent to 1 cup sugar
1/4 cup fresh lemon juice
2/3 cup fresh orange juice

Combine first four ingredients and bring to a boil. Reduce heat; simmer a few minutes, then remove from heat. Add juices and salt. Chill. Serve very cold.

*OLGA'S MINTY DRINK

Exchanges per serving: 1 cup = 1 fruit.
Calories per serving: 40   Yield: 8 cups

1/4 cup mint leaves, chopped fine
Non-nutritive sweetener equivalent to 1/2 cup sugar

1 cup water
1/2 cup fresh lemon juice
2 cups fresh orange juice
4 cups low-calorie ginger ale

Combine first three ingredients and bring to a boil. Cool and strain. When ready to serve, add remaining ingredients and pour over crushed ice in chilled glasses.

*YUMMY COFFEE DRINK

Exchanges per serving: 1 cup = 2 fat.
Calories per serving: 90   Yield: 4 1/2 cups

2 cups strong iced coffee
Non-nutritive sweetener
  equivalent to 1/3 cup sugar

1/2 cup nondairy whipping
  cream
2 cups low-calorie ginger ale

Mix coffee and sweetener. Fill 4 large glasses about 1/4 full with crushed ice. Whip cream. Add 1/4 cup cream and 1/4 cup coffee mixture, then 1/2 cup ginger ale. Stir slightly.

*NONALCOHOLIC EGGNOG

Exchanges per serving: 1 cup = 1/3 skim milk, 1/2 meat.
Calories per serving: 62   Yield: 4 cups

1/2 cup (2 medium) eggs
1/2 cup dry nonfat instant
  powdered milk
2 2/3 cups water, ice cold

Non-nutritive sweetener
  equivalent to 2 tablespoons
  sugar
3 teaspoons vanilla

1 teaspoon rum flavoring

Mix all ingredients well, pour into cups and serve.

*LEMONADE

Exchanges per serving: 1/2 cup = 1/2 fruit.
Calories per serving: 20   Yield: 2 cups

2/3 cup unsweetened lemon
  juice
1 1/2 cups cold water

Sugar syrup substitute
Lemon slices

Combine lemon juice and water. Sweeten with sugar syrup substitute, and add ice. Pour into large glasses on top of ice. Garnish with lemon slice.

*COLA DRINK

Exchanges per serving: 1 cup = 1 skim milk.
Calories per serving: 75   Yield: 2 cups

2 sugarfree, non-caloric cola
  tablets
2 cups skim milk

Non-nutritive sweetener
  equivalent to 1 teaspoon
  sugar

Mix all ingredients well until tablets dissolve.

*CRANBERRY PUNCH

Exchanges per serving: 1/2 cup = 1/2 fruit.
Calories per serving: 20   Yield: 15 cups

8 cups low-calorie cranberry juice cocktail
3 cups unsweetened pineapple juice

Non-nutritive sweetener equivalent to 1/3 cup sugar
4 cups low-calorie ginger ale

Combine juices and sweetener. Chill and stir in ginger ale, which has been well chilled, just before serving; add ice cubes.

*IMITATION WINE

Exchanges per serving: 1/2 cup = 1/2 fruit.
Calories per serving: 20   Yield: 8 cups

2 cups unsweetened grape juice
Non-nutritive sweetener equivalent to 1/3 cup sugar

2 cups low-calorie fruit carbonated beverage, chilled
4 cups low-calorie ginger ale, chilled

Combine juice and sweetener and chill. Stir in carbonated beverage and ginger ale just before serving. Add ice cubes.

*JOAN'S FRUIT SHAKE

Exchanges per serving: 1 cup = 1 fruit, 1/2 skim milk.
Calories per serving: 80   Yield: 4 cups

2 bananas
3 tablespoons fresh orange juice
1/16 teaspoon salt

Non-nutritive sweetener equivalent to 1/2 cup sugar
1/8 teaspoon vanilla
2 cups skim milk

Blend all ingredients until smooth and foamy. Place in refrigerator until chilled, then serve.

*COFFEE PUNCH

Exchanges per serving: 1 cup = 1/4 milk.
Calories per serving: 45   Yield: 24 6-ounce cups

2 cups skim milk
8 cups strong coffee, cold
2 teaspoons vanilla
Non-nutritive sweetener equivalent to 1/2 cup sugar

4 cups ice milk (vanilla, chocolate, or coffee)
1 cup nondairy cream, whipped
1/16 teaspoon cinnamon or nutmeg

Combine milk, coffee, vanilla, and sweetener in large pitcher; stir until sweetener dissolves, then chill. Place chunks of ice milk in punch bowl just before serving. Add coffee mix, put nondairy whipped cream on top, stir lightly; add cinnamon or nutmeg.

*COCOA

Exchanges per serving: 1 cup = 1 skim milk.
Calories per serving: 75   Yield: 8 cups

6 tablespoons unsweetened cocoa
1/2 teaspoon salt
2 cups water

6 cups skim milk
Non-nutritive sweetener equivalent to 1/2 cup sugar

Mix cocoa, salt, and water. Stir constantly over very low heat for 2 minutes. Add milk and sweetener; continue stirring until cocoa again boils; serve.

**WINE LEMONADE

(Not for diabetics without consent of doctor.)

Exchanges per serving: 1 cup = 1/2 fruit.
Calories per serving: 20 + alcohol (approx. 148)   Yield: 6 cups

3 cups water
1/2 cup fresh lemon juice
2 cups white wine

Non-nutritive sweetener equivalent to 1/2 cup sugar

Combine all ingredients and pour over crushed ice in chilled glasses.

**EGGNOG DEVINE

(Not for diabetics without consent of doctor.)

Exchanges per serving: 1/2 cup = 1/2 meat, 1 skim milk.
Calories per serving: 116 + alcohol   Yield: 4 cups

3/4 cup (3 medium) eggs, separated
4 cups skim milk

Non-nutritive sweetener equivalent to 1/2 cup sugar
1/2 cup rum

Beat egg yolks until thick and lemony and combine all ingredients except whites of eggs. Beat whites until stiff and fold in carefully just before serving.

****CHAMPAGNE PUNCH

(Not for diabetics without consent of doctor.)

Exchanges per serving: 1 cup = 1/4 fruit.

Calories per serving: 10 + alcohol (approx. 1246)   Yield: 50 cups

1 Fifth bottle white rum
Non-nutritive sweetener
   equivalent to 1/2 cup sugar
2 cups fresh peaches, sliced
   thin

1/2 cup orange-flavored liqueur
6 Fifth bottles champagne,
   chilled

The day before serving, place rum in bowl; stir in sugar substitute; add peaches as you slice, to prevent their turning brown. Just before serving stir in the orange liqueur; pour over ice in a large punch bowl, add champagne, and serve at once.

SOUPS

Many soup companies can help you plan meals using as a base one of their products. On these you can generally obtain 3 servings per can, with 1 serving equalling 7 ounces (except where noted). If you make the soup with milk, you must, of course, subtract that amount of milk from what is allotted you for that meal. The following, through the courtesy of the Campbell Soup Company, are examples. There are, of course, other varieties manufactured.

PROXIMATE COMPOSITION OF
CAMPBELL SOUP COMPANY PRODUCTS
(Contents of 100 grams, undiluted)*

VARIETY	Cal- ories	Pro- tein	Fat	Car- bohy- drate	So- dium	Vita- min A
Heat Processed Soups		gm	gm	gm	mg	I. U.
Asparagus, Cream of......	70	1.9	2.8	9.4	890	321
Bean with Bacon	133	6.8	4.2	17.1	750	550
Beef..	87	8.0	2.0	9.2	773	1067
Beef Broth	22	3.6	0.0	2.1	708	trace
Beef Noodle	58	3.2	1.9	7.2	795	52
Black Bean..................	80	4.7	1.4	12.2	860	258
Celery, Cream of..........	66	1.4	3.9	6.4	860	173

(*) 100 grams are equivalent to 3 1/2 ounces of 1/3 can of soup. This makes one serving when prepared according to the directions on the label. If soup is prepared with milk, add the nutrients listed opposite the type of milk used. No nutrients are added if soup is prepared with water.

Cheddar Cheese	142	4.8	9.9	8.3	780	300
Chicken Broth...............	36	5.5	1.0	1.2	785	0
Chicken, Cream of.........	76	2.8	4.4	6.3	800	484
Chicken Gumbo.............	49	2.2	1.1	7.5	900	˙179
Chicken 'n Dumplings.....	83	5.8	4.8	4.2	860	175
Chicken Noodle	55	3.3	1.6	6.9	870	47
Chicken with Rice	43	2.8	1.3	4.9	756	133
Chicken and Stars..........	50	3.4	1.3	6.1	930	139
Chicken Vegetable	60	3.4	1.8	7.6	820	2078
Chili Beef	131	6.2	3.7	18.3	860	617
Clam Chowder (Manhattan						
Style)	63	1.9	2.1	9.2	720	713
Consommé...................	28	4.7	0.0	2.5	550	trace
Golden Mushroom	70	2.9	3.5	6.8	840	1170
Green Pea....................	116	6.9	1.6	18.5	760	206
Hot Dog Bean	153	8.4	5.3	18.0	805	510
Minestrone...................	72	3.5	2.4	9.2	788	2167
Mushroom, Cream of......	115	1.7	8.7	7.5	842	79
Noodles and Ground						
Beef.........................	80	3.6	3.7	8.1	760	470
Onion	37	3.5	1.4	2.7	810	trace
Oyster Stew.................	57	1.8	3.2	5.3	780	trace
Pepper Pot...................	83	6.1	3.2	7.6	1000	478
Potato, Cream of...........	59	1.4	1.9	9.0	914	trace
Scotch Broth	74	4.6	2.4	8.6	1000	1867
Split Pea with Ham........	141	10.2	2.6	19.1	803	480
Tomato	69	1.4	1.6	12.3	810	946
Tomato, Bisque of.........	101	2.2	2.1	18.4	870	695
Tomato Rice, Old-						
Fashioned	87	1.6	2.5	14.7	662	917

Turkey Noodle	63	3.3	2.6	6.6	760	120
Turkey Vegetable...........	64	2.7	2.8	7.0	710	2572
Vegetable.....................	68	2.7	1.4	11.1	730	2579
Vegetable Beef	66	5.0	2.3	6.4	755	2795
Vegetable and Beef Stockpot..................	79	4.5	3.4	7.5	785	3235
Vegetable, Old Fashioned	53	2.2	1.7	7.2	713	2242
Vegetarian Vegetable......	62	1.8	1.5	10.4	594	2494

FROZEN SOUPS

Clam Chowder (New England Style)	108	3.7	6.4	8.9	870	50
Green Pea with Ham......	109	7.6	2.3	14.5	750	185
Oyster Stew..................	102	4.6	6.3	6.9	680	191
Potato, Cream of..........	90	2.7	4.3	10.1	944	345
Shrimp, Cream of..........	132	4.0	9.9	6.9	860	93
Vegetable with Beef, Old-Fashioned	68	5.4	2.3	6.6	856	2272

CONDENSED SOUPS IN EXCHANGE LISTS FOR DIABETICS AND OTHER PATIENTS

The following recommendations have been developed by Campbell Soup Company, based on the Standard Exchange Units set forth by American Dietetic Association, American Diabetic Association, and Public Health Service, Department of Health, Education and Welfare.

RECOMMENDATIONS FOR PLACING CAMPBELL'S SOUPS INTO EXCHANGE LISTS

These recommendations are based on a 100-gram portion, which is equivalent of 3 1/2 ounces or 1/3 can of soup. This makes a 7-ounce serving when prepared according to directions on the label. If milk is used in the preparation, use part of your daily allotment. NOTE: When serving a portion, be sure the soup is well blended.

Exchange Substitution for 1
Bread and 1/2 Fat

Frozen Green Pea with Ham
Green Pea
Tomato, Bisque of

Exchange Substitution for 1
Bread

Black Bean
Tomato
Tomato Rice, Old-Fashioned
Vegetable

Exchange Substitution for 1/2
Bread and 1 Fat

Celery, Cream of
Chicken, Cream of
Minestrone
Frozen Potato, Cream of

Exchange Substitution for 1
Meat and 1 Bread

Split Pea with Ham

Exchange Substitution for 1/2
Meat and 1/2 Bread

Beef Soup
Chicken Vegetable
Clam Chowder, Manhattan
Style
Noodles and Ground Beef
Pepper Pot
Scotch Broth
Vegetable Beef
Frozen Vegetable with Beef,
Old-Fashioned

Exchange Substitution for 1/2
Bread and 1/2 Fat

Asparagus, Cream of
Beef Noodle
Chicken Gumbo
Chicken Noodle
Chicken and Stars
Potato, Cream of
Turkey Noodle
Turkey Vegetable
Vegetarian Vegetable
Vegetable, Old-Fashioned

*JOAN'S JELLIED TOMATO CONSOMME

Exchanges per serving: 2/3 cup = 1 fat, 1/2 fruit, 1 "A" vegetable.
Calories per serving: 65 . Yield: 3 cups

1 envelope unflavored gelatin
2 1/4 cups tomato juice
1 bouillon cube, any flavor
1/2 teaspoon salt
Non-nutritive sweetener
 equivalent to 1/4 cup sugar

1/2 teaspoon Worcestershire
 sauce
1/8 teaspoon Tabasco sauce
2 tablespoons lemon juice
1/4 cup cucumbers, unpeeled
 and diced

1/2 cup imitation sour cream
(optional)

Sprinkle gelatin over half the tomato juice in a saucepan. Add bouillon
cube and place over low heat, stirring constantly until gelatin and cube
are dissolved (about 3 minutes). Remove from heat. Add rest of tomato
juice, salt, sweetener, Worcestershire and Tabasco sauces, cucumbers,
and lemon juice. Pour into 2" x 8" x 8" pan and chill until firm. Spoon
into serving dishes. Serve with imitation sour cream topping, if desired.

*ASPARAGUS SOUP

Exchanges per serving: 1/2 cup = No exchange necessary.
Calories per serving: 0   Yield: 5 cups

2 cups asparagus	1/16 teaspoon thyme
3 cups water	1/8 teaspoon salt
4 bouillon cubes, any flavor	1/16 teaspoon pepper

Puree asparagus. Boil water and combine with bouillon cubes, thyme, salt, and pepper. Add asparagus and simmer 5 minutes.

*CUCUMBER SOUP

Exchanges per serving: 1 cup = 1 1/2 fat, 1 "A" vegetable.
Calories per serving: 68   Yield: 3 cups

2 beef or chicken bouillon cubes	1/4 teaspoon lemon peel, dried
2 cups water	1/16 teaspoon seasoned salt
1 cucumber, sliced	1/16 teaspoon pepper
1/2 cup imitation sour cream	1/16 teaspoon thyme

Bring bouillon, water, and cucumber slices to boil. Cover and simmer until tender (about 10 minutes). Cool and place in refrigerator. When cold, blend and add sour cream, lemon peel, and condiments. Blend until smooth. Serve cold.

*VEGETABLE SOUP, COLD
(Gazpacho)

Exchanges per serving: No exchange necessary.
Calories per serving: 0   Yield: 6 servings

1 cup tomatoes, peeled and finely chopped	1 small clove garlic (minced or run through garlic press)
1/2 cup green pepper, finely chopped	3 tablespoons tarragon wine vinegar
1/2 cup celery, finely chopped	1 teaspoon garlic salt
1/2 cup cucumber, peeled and finely chopped	1/4 teaspoon pepper
1/4 cup green onion, finely chopped	1 teaspoon Worcestershire sauce
2 teaspoons parsley, snipped	2 cups tomato juice
1 teaspoon chives, snipped	Hot sauce to taste (approximately 2 teaspoons)

Combine ingredients in either a glass or stainless steel bowl. Take half the mixture and put through blender. When thoroughly blended return to bowl; mix well. Cover bowl and place in refrigerator to chill at least 4 hours, and serve in chilled cups. This may also be used in place of a salad.

*GREAT CARROT or BEAN SOUP

Exchanges per serving: 1 cup carrot = 1 "B" vegetable.
                      1 cup bean = 1 "A" vegetable.
Calories per serving: Carrots, 20; Beans, 0   Yield: 4 cups

1 cup water
2 bouillon cubes, any flavor
2 scant cups carrots (or green
    beans, if preferred)

1/4 teaspoon thyme
1/16 teaspoon salt
1/16 teaspoon pepper

Heat water with bouillon cubes in saucepan and stir occasionally. Add carrots and puree until smooth. Add thyme, salt, and pepper.

*TARRAGON-THYME SOUP

Exchanges per serving: 2/3 cup = 1 fat, 1 "A" vegetable.
Calories per serving: 45   Yield: 2 1/3 cups

2 tablespoons onion, chopped
2 tablespoons celery, chopped
    very fine
1 tablespoon diet margarine
2 cups tomato juice

1/2 teaspoon dried tarragon
1/2 teaspoon salt
1/8 teaspoon pepper
1/16 teaspoon Tabasco sauce,
    if desired

Sauté onion and celery in margarine until onion is golden, then add rest of ingredients. Bring to a boil. Lower heat and simmer 5 minutes.

*EASY PEANUT SOUP

Exchanges per serving: 2/3 cup = 1 bread, 1/2 meat.
Calories per serving: 100   Yield: 4 3/4 cups

1 1/2 cups condensed cream
    of chicken soup
1 1/2 cups cream of celery
    soup

1/4 cup chunky peanut butter
1 1/2 cups water

Blend all ingredients well; let simmer 5 minutes.

**POTATO AND WATERCRESS SOUP

Exchanges per serving: 1 cup = 1/2 bread, 1/2 milk.
Calories per serving: 120   Yield: 3 1/3 cups

1 1/3 cups cream of potato
    soup
1 1/3 cups skim milk
1/2 cup watercress, chopped
    fine (packed tightly)

1/2 teaspoon thyme
1/16 teaspoon salt
1/16 teaspoon pepper

Heat cream of potato soup with skim milk in saucepan. Puree watercress and thyme. Mix with soup until well blended. Add salt and pepper. Cover. Cook and serve hot or cold.

**CELERY BEAN SOUP

Exchanges per serving: 1 cup = 1/2 fat, 1/2 skim milk,
                      1/2 "A" vegetable.

Calories per serving: 98   Yield: 4 cups

1 cup string beans, cut fine
2 tablespoons onion, chopped
  fine
1 1/4 cups cream of celery
  soup

1/16 teaspoon salt
2/3 teaspoon arrowroot powder
1 1/2 cups skim milk

Combine beans and onion with 1/8 cup water, the soup, and half the
salt. Cook in tightly covered saucepan about 6-7 minutes, until onions
soften. In another saucepan combine remaining salt and arrowroot
powder; stir in skim milk gradually to make a smooth mixture. Add to
first mixture and cook over low heat, stirring occasionally until
thickened.

**FESTIVE TOMATO SOUP

Exchanges per serving: 1 scant cup = 1 bread, 1 fruit.
Calories per serving: 110   Yield: 5 2/3 cups

2 2/3 cups tomato soup (do
  not add water)

2/3 cup unsweetened orange
  juice concentrate
2 1/2 cups water

Put tomato soup in pan, add mixture of orange juice and water. Boil
gently. Serve hot or cold.

***SHRIMP CHOWDER

Exchanges per serving: 1/2 cup = 1 bread, 2 meat,
                      1/2 skim milk, 1 "B" vegetable.
Calories per serving: 288   Yield: 8 1/4 cups

1/2 cup onion, finely chopped
1 tablespoon diet margarine
2 cups water
2 teaspoons salt
1 1/4 cups potatoes, pared
  and cubed (about 1/2"
  thick)

2 cups skim milk, scalded
1 2/3 cups shrimp, drained
  and shelled
1/2 tablespoon arrowroot
  powder
1 tablespoon water
1/6 teaspoon salt
1/16 teaspoon pepper

Sauté onion in margarine until golden. Add water, salt, and potatoes.
Boil gently, covered, until potatoes are tender (about 20 minutes). Add
scalded skim milk and shrimp, stirring occasionally. Bring to boil,
reduce heat and simmer until shrimp are pink and cooked (about 5
minutes). Make smooth thin paste of arrowroot and water; add to first
mixture and stir until slightly thickened. Add pepper and remaining
salt, to taste.

**SPLIT PEA SOUP

Exchanges per serving: 1 cup = 1 1/2 bread, 1/2 "B" vegetable.
Calories per serving: 123   Yield: 6 cups

1 cup green split peas, drained
1 carrot, sliced thin
1 onion, sliced thin
5 cups water

3 beef or chicken bouillon cubes
1 teaspoon salt
1/16 teaspoon pepper

1 teaspoon curry powder (optional)

Mix everything except the curry powder together in saucepan. Cover and boil gently until peas are very soft (about 3/4 hour). Stir in curry powder; press mixture through sieve and return puree to saucepan. Reheat and serve.

***TURKEY-WATERCRESS SOUP

Exchanges per serving: 1 cup = 3 meat, 1 "A" and 1 "B" vegetable.
Calories per serving: 260   Yield: 3 cups

1 cup water
1 1/3 cups turkey broth, condensed
2 tablespoons onion, chopped fine
1/4 cup celery, chopped fine
1/2 teaspoon salt

1 1/2 cups cooked turkey, cut in small pieces
1 cup watercress, packed firm (chopped fine)
1 1/2 teaspoons arrowroot powder
2 tablespoons water

Simmer first six ingredients about 15 minutes. Add watercress and simmer again until watercress is wilted. Mix arrowroot powder and two tablespoons water into a smooth paste and stir into soup. Cook until clear and smooth (a few minutes).

***QUICK AND TASTY CHICKEN SOUP

Exchanges per serving: 1 cup = 3 meat.
Calories per serving: 277   Yield: 4 cups

1 1/2 cups chicken or turkey, cooked and diced
1 1/3 cups chicken or turkey broth
1 cup water
2 tablespoons onion, chopped fine

1/4 cup celery, diced fine
1/2 teaspoon salt
1/2 teaspoon thyme
1/2 tablespoon arrowroot powder
1 tablespoon water

Simmer first seven ingredients for about 10 minutes. Make paste with arrowroot and water; add to soup. Cook until clear and smooth (takes just a few seconds).

SALADS

*CUCUMBER SALAD, SWEET AND SOUR

Exchanges per serving: 1/2 cup = 1 "A" vegetable.
Calories per serving: 0

Yield: 2 cups

1/2 cup water
1 cup cider vinegar
Non-nutritive sweetener
equivalent to 1/8 cup sugar
1 stalk celery, sliced thin

1/8 cup dill pickle, chopped
fine
1 1/2 teaspoons salt
2 cucumbers, sliced thin

Boil the water, vinegar, sweetener, pickle, and salt. Place cucumbers and celery slices in glass jar; pour boiling liquid over them, cover and refrigerate overnight. Drain before serving.

*MARINATED VEGETABLE TOSS

Exchanges per serving: 1/2 cup = 1 "A" vegetable.
Calories per serving: 0 (exclusive of dressing)

Yield: 8 servings

2 cups fresh tomato wedges,
peeled
1/2 cup radishes, sliced
1/2 cucumber chunks

1/2 medium red onion, thinly
sliced
1/2 cup celery crescents

Combine all vegetables in salad bowl, pour Italian dressing over. Refrigerate overnight.

*SWEET AND SOUR BEETS

Exchanges per serving: 1 serving = 1/2 meat, 1 "A" and 1 "B"
vegetable.
Calories per serving: 70

Yield: 6 servings

4 cups sliced beets (reserve
juice)
Non-nutritive sweetener
equivalent to 3 tablespoons
sugar
1 teaspoon salt

1/4 teaspoon black pepper
1 tablespoon allspice
1/2 cup vinegar
3 eggs, hard-boiled and shelled
Lettuce

Mix 1/2 cup beet juice with sweetener, salt, pepper, and allspice. Boil gently about 5 minutes. Strain, stir in vinegar. Place eggs and beet slices in baking dish. Pour beet-juice mixture over them and refrigerate overnight, turning both beets and eggs occasionally. Slice eggs with egg slicer; drain beets and divide into 6 servings; place on lettuce leaves. Top each with liquid, then sliced half egg.

*RADISH CELERY SALAD

Exchanges per serving: 1/2 cup = 1 "A" vegetable.
Calories per serving: 0 (exclusive of dressing)   Yield: 2 cups

1 bunch radishes, sliced thin   1/4 cup French dressing (low-
1 cup celery, sliced thin   calorie)
                     Lettuce leaves

Toss radishes, celery, and dressing together. Refrigerate an hour or so before placing on lettuce leaves.

*TOMATO AND HERB SALAD

Exchanges per serving: 1 serving = 1 "A" vegetable.
Calories per serving: 0   Yield: 6 servings

6 tomatoes, peeled   4 tablespoons malt vinegar
1 1/2 teaspoons oregano   1/2 teaspoon seasoned salt
Non-nutritive sweetener   1/4 teaspoon pepper
   equivalent to 1 tablespoon   Lettuce leaves
   sugar

Chop 1 1/2 tomatoes fine; combine with oregano, sweetener, vinegar, and salt. Slice remaining tomatoes, place on top of lettuce leaves; top with vinegar mix; refrigerate until ready to serve.

*PEPPER SLAW

Exchanges per serving: 1/2 cup = 1 "A" vegetable.
Calories per serving: 0 (exclusive of dressing)   Yield: 3 cups

1/2 head cabbage   1/4 green pepper, chopped
1 carrot, chopped fine   fine
                    2 cups water

Cut cabbage into small wedges. Place half in blender along with carrot and pepper. Blend quickly; turn off and drain at once, using liquid for blending with balance of cabbage. Mix with salad dressing.

*MOLDED VEGETABLE SALAD

Exchanges per serving: 1/2 cup = 1 "A" vegetable.
Calories per serving: 10 (+ 9 calories in gelatin)   Yield: 4 servings

1 envelope diet orange gelatin   1/2 cup carrots, shredded
2 cups boiling water   1/4 cup celery, finely chopped
1/2 cup white cabbage,   1/4 teaspoon celery seeds
   chopped

Dissolve gelatin in boiling water. Chill until consistency of egg whites. Fold in vegetables and celery seeds. Pour in pan or molds and refrigerate until firm.

*RASPBERRY RHUBARB SALAD

Exchanges per serving: 1/2 cup = 1/8 fruit.
Calories per serving: 5 (exclusive of dressing)   Yield: 2 cups

1 cup boiling water
1 envelope dietetic raspberry
  gelatin
1/2 cup artificially sweetened
  rhubarb sauce
1/2 teaspoon anise seed,
  crushed fine

1/2 cup apples, chopped fine
1/2 cup celery, chopped fine
1 or 2 drops red vegetable
  coloring
Lettuce

Dissolve gelatin in water. Add rhubarb and anise seed, mix well, and
cool until congealed slightly. Add apples and celery; mix well. Pour into
slightly oiled salad mold and chill until firm. Divide equally on lettuce
and serve with fruit salad dressing, if desired.

*CUCUMBER-PINEAPPLE-GELATIN SALAD

Exchanges per serving: 1/2 cup = 1/2 fruit.
Calories per serving: 20   Yield: 3 1/2 cups

1 envelope diet lemon or
  orange-flavored gelatin
1/2 cup hot water
1/4 cup liquid, drained from
  pineapple tidbits
1/4 cup lemon or orange juice

1/8 teaspoon salt
1 cup artificially sweetened
  dietetic pineapple tidbits
1 1/2 cups cucumber,
  shredded and drained

Dissolve gelatin in hot water. Add pineapple liquid, orange or lemon
juice, and salt. Chill until thickened and consistency of syrup. Then fold
in pineapple and cucumber. Pour into mold and chill.

*LAURA'S JELLIED VEGETABLE SALAD

Exchanges per serving: 1 serving = 1 "A" vegetable.
Calories per serving: 20   Yield: 8 servings

2 envelopes unflavored gelatin
1/2 cup cold water
3 cups boiling water
1/2 cup fresh lemon juice
Non-nutritive sweetener
  equivalent to 2/3 cup sugar

1 tablespoon tarragon vinegar
1 teaspoon salt
3 drops food coloring
1/2 cucumber, diced fine
8-9 radishes, sliced
8-9 scallions, sliced

Soften gelatin in cold water; add boiling water and stir to dissolve.
Blend in lemon juice, sweetener, vinegar, salt, and coloring; chill until
mixture begins to thicken. Fold in vegetables and place in a lightly oiled
mold. Chill until set.

*CARROT SLICES

Exchanges per serving: 2/3 cup = 1/2 bread, 1 "B" vegetable.
Calories per serving: 70   Yield: 3 cups

2 cups carrots, scraped and
   cut into 1" slices
3/4 cup water
1/4 cup cider vinegar
1/2 teaspoon dill pickle,
   chopped fine
1 tablespoon green onion seasoning

1/2 teaspoon poultry seasoning
1/2 teaspoon thyme
1/4 teaspoon garlic salt
1/2 teaspoon marjoram
1/2 teaspoon seasoned salt
1/16 teaspoon lemon pepper
1 cup prepared croutons

Simmer first nine ingredients covered, until carrots are tender. Add salt, pepper, and croutons. Cool. Place in refrigerator for an hour, drain, and serve.

*GOLDEN GLOW SALAD

Exchanges per serving: 1/2 cup = 1 fruit, 1 "A" and 1 "B" vegetable.
Calories per serving: 75   Yield: 4 cups

1 envelope unflavored gelatin
1/8 cup lemon juice
2 cups artificially sweetened
   pineapple tidbits (reserve
   syrup)

1/4 teaspoon salt
1 tablespoon vinegar
1 cup carrots, grated
1/2 cup boiling water
Lettuce

Mix gelatin, lemon juice, and syrup from pineapple tidbits. Soften a few minutes; stir in salt, vinegar, carrots, pineapple, and boiling water. Pour into loaf pan and refrigerate until firm (about 4-5 hours). Serve on lettuce leaves.

*APPLE-CELERY-CRANBERRY-NUT MOLD

Exchanges per serving: 3/4 cup = 1 fat, 1 fruit.
Calories per serving: 85   Yield: 4 1/4 cups

2 cups cranberries
1 1/4 cups water
Non-nutritive sweetener
   equivalent to 1 cup sugar
1 package unflavored gelatin

1 cup apples, peeled and diced
1/2 cup celery, chopped fine
1/2 cup pecans, chopped very
   fine
Lettuce

Cook cranberries in 1 cup water. When skins are broken rub through sieve. Add sweetener and reheat. Soften gelatin in remaining 1/4 cup water, add to cranberry puree and cool. When mixture starts to thicken add apples, celery, and pecans. Pour into mold. Chill. Serve on lettuce.

*PEACH-Y SALAD

Exchanges per serving: 2/3 cup = 1 fruit, 1 "A" vegetable.
Calories per serving: 40   Yield: 4 cups

4 cups artificially sweetened
  peaches, halved
1 tablespoon vinegar
          Lettuce

2 sticks cinnamon
1/2 teaspoon allspice
1 teaspoon cloves, whole

Mix peaches, vinegar, cinnamon, and allspice. Boil gently 5 minutes. Place in refrigerator 5-6 hours. Drain thoroughly; stick a clove in each peach half; serve on lettuce leaves.

*SUPER SALAD

Exchanges per serving: 1 serving = 1 fruit, 1 "A" and 1 "B" vegetable.
Calories per serving: 75   Yield: 3 1/2 cups

1 cup carrots, grated
2 cups unsweetened pineapple
  tidbits (reserve syrup)
1/4 teaspoon salt
1/2 teaspoon anise seed,
  crushed

1 tablespoon white vinegar
1/2 cup boiling water
1/8 cup lemon juice
1 envelope unflavored gelatin
Lettuce

Mix carrots, pineapple, salt, anise seed, vinegar, and water. Stir together lemon juice, gelatin, syrup from pineapple; let soften, then add to first mixture and pour into lightly oiled salad mold. Refrigerate until firm. Loosen mold in hot water; run table knife along inside edges, invert on lettuce.

*JELLIED APPLESAUCE SALAD

Exchanges per serving: 1/2 cup = 1 fruit, 1 "A" vegetable.
Calories per serving: 40 (+ 9 calories in gelatin)   Yield: 4 servings

1 envelope diet raspberry gelatin
1 3/4 cups boiling water
1 cup water-packed ap-
  plesauce

1/2 cup water-packed crushed
  pineapple, drained
1/2 cup celery, chopped

Dissolve gelatin in hot water. Let cool in refrigerator until the consistency of egg whites. Add fruit and celery; stir well. Pour into pan or molds and refrigerate until set (4-5 hours).

*JELLIED FRUIT SALAD

Exchanges per serving: 2/3 cup = 1/2 fruit.
Calories per serving: 20   Yield: 4 cups

1 envelope low-calorie strawberry gelatin dessert
1 3/4 cups boiling water
1/4 cup fresh lemon juice

Non-nutritive sweetener
  equivalent to 1/2 cup sugar
1 cup fresh peaches, sliced fine
1 cup cantaloupe balls

Dissolve gelatin in boiling water. Add lemon juice and sweetener. Chill until consistency of thick syrup; add fruit. Place in lightly oiled mold and chill until set.

*ANN'S APPLE SALAD

Exchanges per serving: 1/2 cup = 1 1/2 fat, 1/2 fruit,
                        1/4 meat, 1 "A" vegetable.
Calories per serving: 100   Yield: 2 cups

1/2 cup apples, thinly sliced
1/2 cup creamed cottage
  cheese
2 tablespoons salad dressing

1/2 cup carrots, grated
1/2 cup celery, chopped fine
1/16 teaspoon salt
Lettuce

Toss together first six ingredients. Divide mixture and place about 1/2 cup portions on lettuce leaves. Refrigerate before serving.

*SLAW

Exchanges per serving: 1 cup = 1 "A" vegetable.
Calories per serving: 8 (exclusive of dressing)   Yield: 4 cups

1/2 head cabbage
1/2 cup carrots, chopped fine

1/2 cup green pepper,
  chopped fine
2 cups water

Shred cabbage. Place half in blender along with carrots, pepper, and water. Blend quickly; turn off and drain at once, using liquid for blending with balance of cabbage. Mix with salad dressing of your choosing.

*MOLDED BEET-ONION SALAD

Exchanges per serving: 1/2 cup = 1 "B" vegetable.
Calories per serving: 35 (+ 9 calories in gelatin)   Yield: 4 servings

1 envelope black raspberry
  diet gelatin
2 cups boiling water

1 cup shoestring beets, drained
1 small jar cocktail pickled
  onions

Dissolve gelatin in boiling water. Chill until consistency of egg whites. Fold in vegetables. Pour in pan or molds and refrigerate until firm (5-6 hours).

**MARGARET'S GELATIN WITH FRUIT

(Not for diabetics without consent of doctor.)

Exchanges per serving: 1 cup = 4 fruit.

Calories per serving: 160 (+ alcohol)　　　　　　Yield: 6 cups

1 cup unsweetened peaches, sliced and drained
1 cup unsweetened pineapple tidbits, drained
1 1/2 tablespoons unflavored gelatin
1 1/4 cups unsweetened grapefruit juice

Non-nutritive sweetener equivalent to 1 cup sugar
1/2 cup wine
3 drops red food coloring
1 cup fresh orange sections
1 cup seedless grapes
2 medium bananas, sliced
2 pears, pared, cored, and diced

Set aside peaches and pineapple. Using liquid from fruit, soften gelatin. Bring grapefruit juice to a boil; add to softened gelatin. Stir to dissolve gelatin, then add sweetener, wine, and food coloring. Refrigerate 3/4 hour. Place peaches, pineapple, and the other fruit in compote and pour chilled gelatin over them. Refrigerate until gelatin thickens, but do not allow to get too firm.

**FROZEN ORANGE FRUIT SALAD

Exchanges per serving: 1/2 filled orange = 2 fat, 1 fruit.

Calories per serving: 130 (+ whipped topping)　　Yield: 8 servings

4 oranges
3/4 cup cream cheese
1/2 cup diet mayonnaise or salad dressing
1 tablespoon lemon juice
1/4 teaspoon prepared mustard

1/4 teaspoon salt
1 cup unsweetened fruit cocktail or mixed unsweetened fruits
1/4 cup slivered almonds
1/2 cup diet topping, whipped and sweetened

Cut oranges in half and scoop out pulp. Combine cream cheese, mayonnaise, lemon juice, mustard, and salt. Add almonds, drained orange pulp and fruit cocktail. Fold in whipped topping. Heap salad in orange halves and freeze until firm. Wrap individually in foil and keep frozen until needed. Remove from freezer 1/2 hour before serving. Garnish with endive or mint.

**MOTHER'S RAW SPINACH SALAD

Exchanges per serving: 1 cup = 3 1/2 fat, 1 "A" vegetable.
Calories per serving: 158   Yield: 5 servings

2 bunches fresh spinach
1/2 medium red onion, sliced
  thin and ringed
6 slices bacon, chopped and
  fried crisp

1/2 cup diet mayonnaise
1/2 cup wine vinegar
Non-nutritive sweetener
  equivalent to 1/2 cup granulated sugar

Wash spinach thoroughly; cut off stems, crisp. Cut in bite-size pieces in
salad bowl; add onion rings and bacon bits. Combine mayonnaise,
vinegar, and sweetener; mix well in blender or mixer. Pour over greens.
Toss and serve at once.

**HOT POTATO SALAD

Exchanges per serving: 1 cup = 1 bread, 1 meat, 1 "A" vegetable.
Calories per serving: 140   Yield: 4 cups

2 cups potatoes, pared and
  cubed
Water (to cover potatoes)
2 1/2 teaspoons salt
1 onion, chopped fine

1 stalk celery, chopped fine
1/4 cup green pepper,
  chopped fine
1 cup nonfat creamed cottage
  cheese

Lettuce

Place potatoes in water to cover; cook until tender; drain. Toss potato
cubes and rest of ingredients together and mix well. Serve on lettuce
leaves.

***MEAT or SEAFOOD SALAD

Suitable for Salads or Sandwich fillings

Exchanges per serving: 3 tablespoons = 2 fat, 2 meat.
Calories per serving: 236   Yield: 3 cups

2 cups minced meat, shellfish,
  or flaked fish
1 tablespoon green onion,
  minced
1/4 cup celery, minced
1 teaspoon pimiento, minced
1 teaspoon fresh parsley,
  minced, or parsley flakes

1 egg, hard-cooked, chopped
  fine
1 teaspoon capers, minced
1/2-3/4 cup diet mayonnaise
  or diet salad dressing
Salt and pepper to taste
Garlic salt to taste

Combine all ingredients. Mix with mayonnaise or salad dressing; season to taste. Chill.

Suggestions: Serve as sandwich filling with plain bread or toasted bun. Serve as main-plate salad:
1. On bed of chopped lettuce, garnished with "A" vegetables.
2. Stuffed in tomato or avocado.

***SEAFOOD SALAD

Exchanges per serving: 1/2 cup = 2 fat, 2 meat.
Calories per serving: 236

Yield: 2 cups

1/2 pound deveined shrimp, shelled, cooked, chilled, and cut in 2" pieces

1 tablespoon green onion, minced

3 tablespoons diet salad dressing

3 tablespoons diet French dressing

1/2 cup chopped nuts

1 cup nonfat creamed cottage cheese

Lettuce

1 tomato, cut in wedges

1 teaspoon parsley sprigs, chopped fine

Mix first six ingredients. Divide evenly on lettuce leaves, garnish with tomato and parsley.

**CAESAR SALAD

Exchanges per serving: 1 cup = 2 fat, 1 meat, 1 "A" vegetable.
Calories per serving: 185

Yield: 6 servings

1 clove garlic

2 heads romaine lettuce
or
1 head iceberg lettuce

1/4 cup olive oil

Juice of 1 lemon

1/4 cup wine vinegar

1 2-ounce can anchovy fillets, drained and chopped

1/4 cup Parmesan cheese

1/2 cup prepared croutons

1 egg, well beaten

Salt and pepper to taste

Rub salad bowl with cut clove of garlic. Tear cleaned and crisped lettuce into bite-size pieces in salad bowl. Pour olive oil, lemon juice, and vinegar over greens; toss lightly. Sprinkle chopped anchovies, grated cheese, and croutons on top; add beaten egg. Season. Toss and serve at once.

****LOTTIE'S COTTAGE CHEESE MOLD

Exchanges per serving: 1 serving = 1/2 skim milk, 4 meat.
Calories per serving: 332   Yield: 3 servings

2 cups minced clams
1 envelope unflavored gelatin
1 1/4 cups skim milk
1/2 teaspoon Worcestershire sauce
1/2 teaspoon salt
1/16 teaspoon Tabasco sauce
1/16 teaspoon allspice
2/3 cup nonfat cottage cheese
1 tablespoon green pepper, chopped fine
1/2 tablespoon onion, chopped fine

Drain clams, reserve 1/2 cup liquid. Sprinkle gelatin on clam liquid in saucepan to soften; place over low heat and stir until gelatin dissolves (2-3 minutes). Remove from heat. Add milk, Worcestershire sauce, salt, Tabasco and allspice. Chill until mixture has the consistency of unbeaten egg whites. Add clams, cottage cheese, pepper, and onion. Place in small loaf pan and chill until firm. Unmold to serve.

****NUT AND CHEESE SALAD

Exchanges per serving: 3/4 cup = 2 fat, 2 meat, 1 "A" vegetable.
Calories per serving: 336   Yield: 3 cups

2 cups nonfat creamed cottage cheese
1 cup chopped nuts
2 small dill pickles, chopped fine
Lettuce

Mix first three ingredients well and serve on lettuce leaves.

****FISH AND POTATO SALAD

Exchanges per serving: 1 serving = 1 bread, 2 fat, 3 meat, 1 "A" vegetable.
Calories per serving: 377   Yield: 3 servings

3 potatoes
2 cups fish, flaked
2 tablespoons pimiento, chopped
2 tablespoons onion, minced
2 tablespoons parsley, snipped
1 cup celery, sliced thin
1/4 cup vinegar
2 tablespoons salad oil
1 teaspoon salt
1/8 teaspoon pepper
Lettuce

Wash, pare, and slice potatoes thin. Boil gently about 5-6 minutes in salted boiling water to cover until nearly tender. When potatoes are almost done, add fish. Bring water back to boil, cover, and gently boil about 5 minutes. Drain liquid, cool potatoes slightly, then place in refrigerator until serving. Toss remaining ingredients (except lettuce) in large bowl and mix well. Cover and place in refrigerator until time to serve. Add potatoes and fish to dressing; toss and mix. Serve on lettuce leaves.

*EASY SALAD DRESSING

Exchanges per serving: 1 tablespoon = None.
Calories per serving: 0   Yield: 1 1/4 cups

1/4 cup eggs, well beaten
1/2 teaspoon salt
1/16 teaspoon pepper
1/2 teaspoon dry mustard

1/2 cup vinegar
1/2 cup skim milk
Non-nutritive sweetener equivalent to 1/2 cup sugar

Mix all ingredients except sweetener and cook until mixture comes to a racing boil, over low heat. Add sweetener and cool. Use for salads.

*VINEGAR DRESSING

Exchanges per serving: None.
Calories per serving: 0   Yield: 1/3 cup

1/4 cup vinegar
2 tablespoons water
1 clove garlic, crushed
1/8 teaspoon salt
1/8 teaspoon paprika

Non-nutritive sweetener equivalent to 3 1/2 teaspoons sugar
1/2 teaspoon dill or tarragon or a combination of rosemary and thyme

Combine all ingredients. Store in jar in refrigerator. Shake well before using.

*FRUIT SALAD DRESSING

Exchanges per serving: 1 tablespoon = None.
Calories per serving: 5   Yield: 3/4 cup

Non-nutritive sweetener equivalent to 3 cups sugar
1/2 cup unsweetened lemon juice
1/2 cup water
1/2 tablespoon arrowroot powder

1/2 teaspoon celery seed
1/2 teaspoon chervil
1 teaspoon celery salt
1/2 teaspoon dry mustard
1/2 teaspoon paprika

Combine sweetener, lemon juice, water, and arrowroot powder in a small pan and stir to blend. Add rest of ingredients and bring to a boil, cooking until thick and clear (about 3-4 minutes), stirring constantly. Cool, store in refrigerator.

*SKIM MILK DRESSING

Exchanges per serving: 1 tablespoon = None.
Calories per serving: 7   Yield: 3 cups

1 cup white vinegar   2 cups skim milk
Non-nutritive sweetener
equivalent to 3/4 cup sugar

Beat all ingredients thoroughly with rotary beater. Store in refrigerator.
May be used for lettuce, coleslaw, etc.

*SALLY'S SALAD DRESSING

Exchanges per serving: 1 tablespoon = None.
Calories per serving: 8   Yield: 3 ounces or 5 tablespoons

2 teaspoons minced onion   Non-nutritive sweetener
4 tablespoons malt or cider   equivalent to 1/2 cup sugar
vinegar   2 teaspoons seasoned salt
                    1/8 teaspoon lemon pepper

Mix all ingredients well. Serve on fruit or vegetable salads or for
coleslaw mix.

*LOW-CALORIE DRESSING

Exchanges per serving: 2 tablespoons = None.
Calories per serving: 10   Yield: 1 1/2 cups

1 1/4 cups condensed tomato   1/8 teaspoon black pepper
soup, undiluted   1/4 teaspoon garlic powder
1/4 teaspoon onion salt   3 tablespoons wine vinegar
                   1 tablespoon corn relish

Mix all ingredients together in large jar. Cover and refrigerate. Shake
before using.

*MARGE'S SALAD DRESSING

Exchanges per serving: 1 tablespoon = None.
Calories per serving: 10   Yield: 1 1/2 cups

1/4 cup (1 medium) egg, well   1/2 cup malt vinegar
beaten   1 teaspoon mustard
Non-nutritive sweetener   1/2 teaspoon salt
equivalent to 2/3 cup sugar   1/8 teaspoon pepper
2/3 cup skim milk   1/2 teaspoon diet margarine

Combine all ingredients in top of double boiler and cook over hot
water. Stir until thick and smooth. Chill. Use for vegetable salads.

*DRESSING A LA BLANCHE

Exchanges per serving: 1 tablespoon = None.
Calories per serving: 16
Yield: 3 cups

1 cup white vinegar
2 cups skim milk

Non-nutritive sweetener
equivalent to 3/4 cup sugar

Place all ingredients in covered glass jar; shake until well mixed. Store in refrigerator. Use for lettuce, coleslaw, etc.

*FRUIT DRESSING

Exchanges per serving: 1 tablespoon = 1/2 fat.
Calories per serving: 20
Yield: 3 cups

1/4 teaspoon dry mustard
1/4 teaspoon salt
1 teaspoon onion juice
1 cup cider vinegar
4 teaspoons paprika

4 tablespoons celery seed
1 1/2 cups water
1/2 cup oil
Non-nutritive sweetener
equivalent to 3 cups sugar

Combine first five ingredients. Bring to boil. Simmer over low heat about 5 minutes; remove from heat and add remaining ingredients. Chill. Serve on fruit salads.

*LOUISE'S SALAD DRESSING

Exchanges per serving: 1 tablespoon = 1/2 fat.
Calories per serving: 20
Yield: 1 cup

1/4 cup (3 medium) egg yolk,
  beaten well
2 tablespoons skim milk
Non-nutritive sweetener
  equivalent to 1/2 cup sugar

1/2 cup fresh lemon juice
2 teaspoons diet margarine,
  melted
1/8 teaspoon salt

Mix all ingredients in saucepan and cook over medium heat. Stir constantly, until mixture comes to a boil and is slightly thick. Chill.

*GOURMET SOUR CREAM DRESSING

Exchanges per serving: 1 tablespoon = 1 fat.
Calories per serving: 45
Yield: 1 1/4 cups

2 tablespoons green onion,
  minced
3 tablespoons wine vinegar
Non-caloric sweetener equivalent to 2 tablespoons sugar

1 teaspoon salt
1 teaspoon prepared mustard
1/8 teaspoon pepper
Dash of pepper sauce
1 cup sour cream

Combine all ingredients. Chill at least 1/2 hour to blend flavors.

*GINNY'S SALAD DRESSING

Exchanges per serving: 1 tablespoon = None.
Calories per serving: 0   Yield: 5 tablespoons

2 teaspoons onion juice
4 tablespoons cider vinegar
Non-nutritive sweetener
  equivalent to 1/2 cup sugar

1/8 teaspoon dry mustard
1/8 teaspoon pepper
1/8 teaspoon salt

Mix all ingredients well. Serve on fruit or vegetable salads or for
coleslaw mix.

*SALAD DRESSING

Exchange per serving: 1 tablespoon = None.
Calories per serving: 10   Yield: 2 cups

1/2 cup (2 medium) eggs, well
  beaten
1 teaspoon salt
1/8 teaspoon lemon pepper
1 teaspoon dry mustard

1 cup malt or cider vinegar
1 cup skim milk
Non-nutritive sweetener
  equivalent to 1 cup sugar

Mix first six ingredients. Cook until mixture comes to a racing boil,
over low heat. Add sweetener; cool.

*CHUTNEY AND CURRY MAYONNAISE

Exchanges per serving: 1 tablespoon = 1 fat.
Calories per serving: 45   Yield: 1 cup

1 cup safflower mayonnaise
1 teaspoon any minced fruit

1 teaspoon chutney or curry
powder

Blend all ingredients together for spicy sauce for seafoods and chicken
salad.

*FRENCH VINEGAR STYLE DRESSING

Exchanges per serving: 1 tablespoon = 1 1/2 fat.
Calories per serving: 65   Yield: 3/4 cup

2 tablespoons vinegar
1/2 teaspoon salt
1 teaspoon paprika
4 tablespoons lemon juice

1/2 onion, grated fine
6 tablespoons oil
Non-nutritive sweetener
  equivalent to 1 cup sugar

Bring vinegar, salt, paprika, lemon juice, and onion to a boil. Cool. Add
oil and sweetener and cook until thick as desired.

*BLEU CHEESE TOPPING

Exchanges per serving: 1 tablespoon = None.
Calories per serving: 19   Yield: 2 1/4 cups

2 cups unflavored low-calorie   3 tablespoons low-calorie bleu
   yogurt   cheese dressing
                      1/2 teaspoon salt

Combine ingredients, then chill. Serve on lettuce leaves.

*THOUSAND ISLAND DRESSING

Exchanges per serving: 1 tablespoon = None.
Calories per serving: 23   Yield: 1 1/3 cups

1 cup unflavored low-calorie   1 tablespoon onion, chopped
   yogurt   fine
1/4 cup low-calorie catsup   Non-nutritive sweetener
2 tablespoons celery, diced   equivalent to 1/2 cup sugar
   fine   1/4 teaspoon seasoned salt
1 tablespoon green pepper,   1/4 teaspoon pepper
   diced fine

Mix all ingredients and blend well. Chill overnight in refrigerator.

*LUAU MAYONNAISE

Exchanges per serving: 1 ounce = 1 1/2 fat.
Calories per serving: 80   Yield: 1 1/4 cups

1 cup safflower mayonnaise   1 tablespoon maraschino cher-
2 tablespoons artificially   ry syrup
   sweetened pineapple juice

Thin mayonnaise with juice and syrup and blend to smooth pink color.

*DOTTIE'S FRENCH DRESSING

Exchanges per serving: 1 tablespoon = 2 fat.
Calories per serving: 90   Yield: 3/4 cup

1/2 cup olive oil   1 teaspoon salt
1/4 cup malt vinegar   1/16 teaspoon paprika
1/4 teaspoon dry mustard   1/16 teaspoon lemon pepper

Place all ingredients in glass jar. Blend or shake until well mixed. Chill.

CHEESE AND EGG DISHES

Fried eggs and omelets can be cooked beautifully in a Teflon-coated pan without the addition of fat.

When using basic ingredients such as arrowroot, eggs, flour, margarine, and tapioca, refer to General Information and to Table of Weights and Measures.

*FLUFF OMELET

Exchanges per serving: 1 serving = 1 meat.
Calories per serving: 75

Yield: 1 serving

1/4 cup (1 medium) egg
1 tablespoon water

1/16 tablespoon salt

Using a wire whip, beat all ingredients together. Place in Teflon pan and cook until done.

VARIATIONS: Diet Jelly: No additional calories.
Cheese: 1/2 ounce grated cheese, add 35 calories to above.
Ham and Green Pepper: 20 grams ham and green pepper, chopped, add 35 calories to above.

*SCRAMBLED EGGS

Exchanges per serving: 1 serving = 1 meat.
Calories per serving: 85

Yield: 1 serving

1/4 cup (1 medium) egg
1 tablespoon skim or whole milk

salt
pepper

To eliminate the use of fat, scramble eggs in a double boiler (or use Teflon-coated pan). Mix egg and milk with wire whip or fork; add salt and pepper and for variety, a dash of curry powder or chopped chives, green onion, or parsley. For a marvelous variation, add 2 tablespoons Spanish sauce to raw egg mixture, then cook.

*BLINTZES WITH CHEESE FILLING

Exchanges per serving: 1 blintze = 1/2 bread, 3/4 meat.
Calories per serving: 85   Yield: 1 dozen

1 cup flour
1/2 teaspoon salt
1/2 teaspoon baking powder
1 cup skim milk
3/4 cup (3 medium) eggs
2 tablespoons diet margarine, melted

2 cups low-calorie cottage cheese, sieved
Non-nutritive sweetener equivalent to 2 tablespoons sugar
1/2 teaspoon cinnamon
1/4 teaspoon allspice or nutmeg

Sift flour, salt, and baking powder together. Beat milk, 1/2 cup (2 medium) eggs, and margarine. Slowly add to flour mixture; stir to form thin batter. Grease frying pan lightly, then pour 1/8 cup batter into skillet and cover bottom completely. Cook until top of pancake is bubbly, then turn onto paper towel. Make rest of pancakes, greasing skillet as necessary. Mix cottage cheese, sweetener, cinnamon, allspice or nutmeg, and remaining egg. Top each pancake, which has been turned brown side up, with tablespoon of filling. Fold over sides, then the ends to make small drugstore-type package; set to one side. Refrigerate until ready to serve. A few minutes before serving, melt margarine in skillet and lightly brown each blintze, starting with flap side down. Then turn and brown other side. Serve warm.

**SALLY'S CHEESE FONDUE

(Not for diabetics without consent of doctor.)
Exchanges per serving: 1 slice = 1 bread, 2/3 meat, 1/3 milk.
Calories per serving: 175 (+ wine)   Yield: 12 servings

1 clove garlic, peeled
2 cups dry white wine
2 cups cheese, shredded fine
1/4 teaspoon arrowroot powder
2 tablespoons Kirschwasser (if approved by doctor)

1/16 teaspoon pepper
1/16 teaspoon salt
1/16 teaspoon nutmeg
12 slices bread, cut into cubes leaving one side of crust on each cube

Rub an earthenware casserole with garlic, then add wine. Heat slowly over chafing dish burner. Mix cheese lightly with arrowroot powder; when bubbles in wine rise to surface, add cheese mix a handful at a time. Stir until each handful melts and continue until all cheese is melted; add Kirschwasser and seasonings. Stir well. Turn heat low but keep fondue slowly bubbling. Each person takes a cube of bread on the end of his fork and twirls it in the bubbling fondue. If fondue is too thick, add a little *hot* wine.

**HAM AND CHEESE ON BUNS

Exchanges per serving: 1/2 bun = 1/2 bread, 2 meat.
Calories per serving: 185   Yield: 3 buns

3 buns, cut in half   1/4 cup dietetic cranberry sauce
6 slices ham, baked   6 slices Mozarella cheese

Toast halves of bun slightly, then top with slice of ham. Spread each
with cranberry sauce and place thin slice of cheese over this; put under
broiler until cheese melts and is lightly browned.

**EGGS ON TOAST, OVEN STYLE

Exchanges per serving: 1 serving = 1 bread, 1 fat, 1 meat.
Calories per serving: 190   Yield: 6 servings

6 slices bread   1 tablespoon chervil
6 teaspoons diet margarine   1/8 teaspoon salt
1 1/2 cups (6 medium) eggs,   1/8 teaspoon pepper
    separated

Preheat oven to 350°. Butter each slice of bread with margarine and
place buttered side up on cookie sheet. Beat egg whites until stiff and
distribute evenly on each slice of bread. Make a hollow in center of
white, then fill with yolk. Sprinkle eggs with chervil, salt, and pepper.
Bake until yolk is nearly set and white is lightly browned (about 15
minutes). Serve at once.

***EGGS WITH CHEESE SAUCE

Exchanges per serving: 2/3 cup = 1 1/2 bread,
                              1/2 fat, 2 meat.
Calories per serving: 278   Yield: 4 cups

1 1/4 tablespoons arrowroot   1 tablespoon chervil
    powder   1/2 cup milk
1/2 teaspoon salt   1 tablespoon diet margarine
1/16 teaspoon cayenne   1 1/2 cups cheese, grated fine
1 tablespoon prepared mus-   1 1/2 cups (6 medium) eggs
    tard   6 slices bread

Preheat oven to 350°. Butter individual custard cups. Mix first five
ingredients together. Stir in milk slowly; continue stirring until thick
and smooth, over medium heat. Remove from heat and stir in
margarine and cheese. Stir until cheese has melted and sauce is smooth.
Into each cup break one egg; cover with 1/4 cup cheese sauce and bake
until firm (15-20 minutes). Toast bread, cut in half, and serve egg with
toast.

***CHEESE TOAST AND EGGS

Exchanges per serving: 1 serving = 1 bread, 2 meat.
Calories per serving: 220   Yield: 4 servings

4 slices bread
4 ounces Mozarella cheese

1 cup (4 medium) eggs, poached

Preheat oven to 350°. Toast bread, top with 1/4 of cheese for each slice. Put on cookie sheet and place in oven until cheese just melts (2-3 minutes). Add poached egg on top. Serve at once.

***EGGS CURRY

Exchanges per serving: 1 serving = 1 bread, 1 fat, 1 meat,
                             1 skim milk, 1 "B" vegetable.
Calories per serving: 260   Yield: 4 servings

6 hard-boiled eggs
1/4 cup almonds, slivered
2 tablespoons diet margarine
1 onion, chopped fine
1/2 cup celery, chopped fine

1 1/2 tablespoons arrowroot powder
1 teaspoon salt
1 1/2 teaspoons curry powder
2 cups skim milk
4 slices toast

Thinly slice shelled eggs. Brown almonds in margarine until golden brown. Remove and drain on absorbent paper. In same pan sauté onion and celery until golden, then stir in arrowroot, salt, and curry powder. Stir in milk slowly; cook, stirring constantly until thick and smooth. Stir in sliced eggs and heat to boil. Place a slice of toast in the bottom of each of four, individual, heated casseroles. Divide the eggs evenly over the toast and sprinkle with almonds.

***OMELET WITH COTTAGE CHEESE

Exchanges per serving: 1 serving = 1 fat, 3 meat.
Calories per serving: 270   Yield: 2 servings

2 tablespoons diet margarine
1 cup (4 medium) eggs, separated
1/16 teaspoon salt

1/2 cup low-calorie cottage cheese, sieved
1/16 teaspoon pepper
1 tablespoon chervil

Preheat oven to 350°. Melt margarine in skillet. Beat egg whites and salt until stiff, but not dry. Beat yolks separately until lemon-colored and thick, then add cheese and pepper and beat until smooth. Fold in egg whites and chervil. Place mixture in skillet and cook over medium heat until lightly browned on bottom and fluffy (about 3-4 minutes). Place in oven 15 minutes; make a crease down center with knife and fold over. Serve at once.

****CHEESE FONDUE

Exchanges per serving: 1 serving = 1 bread,
                     3 meat, 1/4 milk.
Calories per serving: 329   Yield: 4 servings

1 cup milk
1 tablespoon diet margarine
1/8 teaspoon pepper
1/4 teaspoon salt
1 1/2 cups bread cubes

2/3 cup cheddar cheese, grated
3/4 cup (3 medium) eggs, separated

Preheat oven to 375°. Place a 2" x 9" x 9" cake pan, filled about 1/2" deep with hot water, in oven. Scald milk, add margarine, pepper, and salt. Stir to melt margarine, then stir in bread cubes and cheese until completely mixed. Add yolks of eggs and stir until smooth. Beat whites of eggs until stiff enough to form peaks. Pour milk-bread mixture over egg whites and fold in gently. Pour into greased casserole; place casserole in water in the cake pan and bake until browned (about 3/4 hour). Serve at once.

FISH, MEAT AND POULTRY

PROXIMATE COMPOSITION OF
CAMPBELL SOUP COMPANY PRODUCTS

(Contents of 100 grams, equivalent to one 3 1/2-ounce can. This makes one serving when prepared according to the directions.)

VARIETY	Cal- ories	Pro- tein	Fat	Car- bohy- drate	So- dium	Vita- min A
Heat Processed Soups		gm	gm	gm	mg	I. U.
Barbecue Beans..............	126	5.7	1.5	22.5	406	225
Beans and Franks..........	160	8.4	7.1	15.7	481	128
Beans and Ground Beef ...	114	7.1	2.7	15.3	500	860
Pork and Beans..............	115	7.1	1.3	18.8	420	113
BOUNTY MAIN DISH PRODUCTS:						
Beef Stew......................	79	7.2	2.5	7.0	440	1923
Chicken Stew................	82	6.1	3.4	6.8	420	1942
Chili Con Carne (with beans)	119	7.0	5.8	9.6	470	583
Chili Mac	114	5.6	4.4	13.0	550	520
Corned Beef Hash	184	11.5	10.6	10.7	650	trace
FRANCO-AMERICAN PRODUCTS:						
Beef Gravy....................	49	3.1	1.9	4.9	562	trace
Chicken Giblet Gravy.....	48	1.8	2.3	4.9	590	490
Chicken Gravy..............	88	2.3	6.3	5.5	480	583
Italian Style Spaghetti	77	3.5	0.9	13.6	432	255

Macaroni with Cheese

Sauce	97	3.7	4.2	11.0	440	228

Macaroni with Cheese

Item						
Sauce	97	3.7	4.2	11.0	440	228
Macaroni 'n Beef	99	5.4	3.7	11.0	610	353
MacaroniO's	75	3.4	2.5	9.8	485	270
Spaghetti with Ground Beef	119	4.9	6.1	11.2	507	750
Spaghetti with Meat- balls........................	116	4.9	6.0	10.7	488	485
Spaghetti with Tomato Sauce	81	3.2	0.7	15.6	403	200
SpaghettiO's.................	81	2.7	1.0	15.2	475	350
SpaghettiO's with Franks	111	3.9	5.6	11.3	577	280
SpaghettiO's with Meatballs.................	94	4.7	3.9	10.1	560	425
Spaghetti Sauce with Meat.......................	96	4.6	5.2	7.9	740	2614
Spaghetti Sauce with Mushrooms..............	77	1.5	3.0	10.9	880	935

OTHER CAMPBELL PRODUCTS IN EXCHANGE LISTS

(100 gram portion measures between 1/3 and 1/2 cup)

Exchange Substitution for 1 1/2 Meat and 1 Bread

Bounty Corned Beef Hash

Exchange Substitution for 1 Meat and 1/2 Bread

Bounty Chili Con Carne

Exchange Substitution for 1/2 Meat and 1 Vegetable "B"

Bounty Beef Stew
Bounty Chicken Stew

Other products that you may serve but do not need to measure are:
Beef Broth
Consommé
Tomato Juice
"V-8" Cocktail Vegetable Juice

** CHOP SUEY WITH TUNA

Exchanges per serving: 1 cup = 1 bread, 1 meat.
Calories per serving: 145

Yield: 4 servings

2 stalks celery, cut small
1/2 onion, chopped fine
2 cups + 2 tablespoons water
3/4 cup rice
Non-nutritive sweetener
  equivalent to 1/2 teaspoon
  sugar

1/6 teaspoon pepper
2 tablespoons soy sauce
3/4 cup water-packed tuna,
  drained

Cook celery and onion in 2 tablespoons water over low heat, covered. When tender, remove from heat; add rice, 2 cups water, and seasonings. Bring to boil. Turn heat to low and cook, covered, until rice is tender and liquid absorbed (about 1/2 hour). Add tuna. Mix and remove from heat. Set aside, covered, for a few minutes before serving.

*** CHEESE AND CRAB ORIENTAL STYLE

Exchanges per serving: 1 serving = 1/4 bread, 2 1/2 meat, 2 "A" and
                        1/4 "B" vegetables.
Calories per serving: 220

Yield: 5 servings

1/2 cup mushrooms, sliced
1/2 carrot, sliced thin
1/4 cup green pepper, diced
1 cup celery, sliced
1 cup onion, chopped fine
2 tablespoons oil
Non-nutritive sweetener
  equivalent to 1 tablespoon
  sugar

1 teaspoon salt
1 bay leaf
4 cups tomatoes
3/4 cup rice, precooked
1 1/2 cups crab meat, frozen,
  thawed, and drained
1/2 cup sharp cheese, grated

Preheat oven to 350°. Sauté first five ingredients in oil in Dutch oven or other oven-proof container until the onion is golden brown. Add sweetener, salt, bay leaf and tomatoes and boil for 5 minutes, gently. Stir in rice and crab meat. Sprinkle entire mixture with grated cheese. Bake 20-25 minutes.

***FISH AND MUSHROOMS

Exchanges per serving: 1 serving = 1 fat, 3 meat,
1 "A" vegetable.

Calories per serving: 260 (plus sherry)   Yield: 4 servings

1 onion, sliced thin
1 tablespoon oil
1 1/2 cups mushrooms, sliced thin
1 pound fish fillets (cod, halibut, sole) cut in 1" slices

1/6 teaspoon salt
1/16 teaspoon pepper
1 stalk celery, sliced thin
1 tablespoon soy sauce
1 tablespoon dry sherry (if permitted by doctor)

Preheat skillet and sauté onion in oil. Add mushrooms and sauté about 2 minutes, stirring all the while, until mushrooms have wilted. Then spread fillet slices on mushrooms; sprinkle with salt and pepper, add remaining fillets, sprinkle these with salt and pepper. Add celery, soy sauce and sherry and cook gently, covered, for ten minutes.

***HARRIET'S FISH DISH

Exchanges per serving: 1 serving = 1/2 fat, 3 meat, 1 "A" and
1 "B" vegetable.

Calories per serving: 270   Yield: 4 servings

2 onions, sliced thin
1 clove garlic, crushed
1 tablespoon diet margarine
1/2 cup parsley, snipped
1/2 teaspoon salt
1/8 teaspoon pepper

2 cups canned tomatoes
1 tablespoon tomato paste
2 chicken bouillon cubes
4 4-ounce fish fillets or steaks
3 slices tomato, cut thin
3 slices lemon, cut thin

Preheat oven to 300°. Sauté onions and garlic in margarine until golden; add parsley, salt, pepper, tomatoes with juice, tomato paste, and bouillon cubes. Simmer gently, uncovered, about 20 minutes. Then place fish steaks, cut about 3/4" thick, in medium baking dish. Cover with sauce, top with slices of tomatoes and lemons. Bake until tender.

***BAKED FISH STEAKS

Exchanges per serving: 3 ounces = 1 fat, 3 meat.
1/4 "B" vegetable.

Calories per serving: 280   Yield: 4 servings

4 3-ounce fish steaks (halibut, swordfish, etc.)
4 tablespoons oil
1 onion, sliced thin

1 potato, sliced thin
1/2 carrot, sliced thin
1/16 teaspoon salt
1/16 teaspoon pepper
1/2 teaspoon parsley, snipped

Preheat oven to 450°. Remove skin from fish steaks and cut meat away from bone. Pour oil in center of a piece of heavy-duty foil and place steaks on oil. Top each piece with slice of onion, potato, carrot, and salt and pepper. Using drugstore folds, wrap each piece separately. Put on cookie sheet and bake until fish flakes easily and is tender. Garnish with parsley.

***HILO FILLET OF SOLE

Exchanges per serving: 3 ounces = 3 fat, 2 meat.
Calories per serving: 275   Yield: 8 servings

1 1/2 pound fish fillets (cod, halibut, sole)
1/4 teaspoon salt
2 teaspoons instant minced onion
1 1/2 teaspoons water
3/4 cup safflower mayonnaise

1 teaspoon lemon juice
1/4 teaspoon seasoned salt
1 teaspoon parsley, finely chopped
1/3 cup macademia nuts, chopped, or slivered almonds

Wipe fillets with a damp cloth. Sprinkle with salt. Roll and secure each with toothpick. Place rolls in steamer or on wire rack above boiling water; cover and steam 15 minutes. Mix onion, water, mayonnaise, lemon juice, seasoned salt, and parsley. Remove fillets carefully from steamer and spread quickly with mayonnaise mixture. Top with nuts and serve at once.

****TASTY FILLETS

Exchanges per serving: 1 serving = 1 fat, 4 meat.
Calories per serving: 320   Yield: 3 servings

1 pound fish fillets
1/2 cup sour cream
1/8 teaspoon ginger
1/8 teaspoon dry mustard
1/8 teaspoon thyme

1/4 teaspoon salt
1/6 teaspoon paprika
1/8 teaspoon parsley, snipped fine

Preheat oven to 400°. Grease 2" x 6" x 10" baking dish. Divide fillets into 3 servings. Sprinkle with salt on both sides and place in baking dish in one layer. Mix sour cream, ginger, mustard, thyme, and salt and spread mixture on top of fillets. Bake until fish is tender and easily flaked (about 20-25 minutes). Top with paprika and parsley. Serve at once.

***SHRIMP AND RICE

Exchanges per serving: 2/3 cup rice and 3/4 cup sauce = 1 bread, 3 meat, 1 "A" vegetable.

Calories per serving: 287   Yield: 5 servings

2 cups tomatoes
2 tablespoons parsley flakes
2 cups celery, sliced thin
1/4 teaspoon basil
1 1/2 teaspoons salt
1/8 teaspoon pepper

1/2 teaspoon oregano
1 3-ounce can tomato paste
1/2 cup long-grain rice
2 7-ounce packages frozen, deveined, shelled shrimp

Mix everything except rice and shrimp in large skillet. Stir occasionally. Boil gently, uncovered, until celery is nearly tender (about 1/2 hour). Stir in shrimp and boil until shrimp are cooked but still tender (about 5-10 minutes). Cook rice as directed, omitting margarine or butter. Serve shrimp over rice.

***CRAB, SHRIMP, RICE SUPREME

Exchanges per serving: 3/4 cup = 1/2 bread, 3 fat, 1 1/3 meat.

Calories per serving: 270   Yield: 8-10 servings

2 cups cooked rice
1 cup diet mayonnaise
1/2 cup green onion, chopped
1/4 cup green pepper, chopped
1 cup tomato juice
1/4 cup toasted almonds, slivered

8-ounce fresh, frozen, or canned crab meat
8-ounce fresh, frozen, or canned shrimp
1/4 cup prepared bread crumbs

Preheat oven to 350°. Mix all ingredients (except bread crumbs) together, place in casserole, top with the bread crumbs. Bake 1 hour. Use fresh seafood if available. This is an excellent party casserole as it can be made a day ahead and refrigerated.

***TUNA (or SALMON) PIE WITH CRUST

Exchanges per serving: 1 serving = 1 bread, 1/2 fat, 3 meat.

Calories per serving: 300   Yield: 6 servings

1 cup long-grain white rice, uncooked
2 tablespoons diet margarine
3/4 cup (3 medium) eggs
1 1/4 cups water-packed tuna (or pink salmon), drained and flaked

1/4 teaspoon salt
1/8 teaspoon pepper
1/8 teaspoon nutmeg
3/4 cup American cheese, grated
3/4 cup skim milk, scalded
1/2 teaspoon parsley

Preheat oven to 400°. Cook rice as directed, then mix with margarine and half the egg. Line a 9" pie pan and mound rice mixture up to about 1" above rim of plate. Spread tuna (or salmon) in shell, sprinkle with salt, pepper, nutmeg, and cheese. Beat remaining egg in small bowl and stir in scalded milk. Heat until smooth, then pour mixture over cheese. Bake until cheese is dark golden brown (about 1/2 hour). Sprinkle parsley over top, if desired.

***SALMON (or TUNA) CASSEROLE

Exchanges per serving: 1/2 cup = 1/2 bread, 1/2 fat, 1/2 milk, 1 1/2 meat.

Calories per serving: 260   Yield: 24 servings

1 cup noodles	1/2 cup flour
2 cups mushrooms, sliced thin	2 teaspoons paprika
4 tablespoons onion, chopped fine	2 cups milk
	2 cups light cream
4 tablespoons diet margarine	4 cups pink salmon (or tuna,
1 teaspoon salt	water-packed and well
1/4 teaspoon pepper	drained)

1 cup Parmesan cheese, grated

Preheat oven to 375°. Cook noodles according to directions on the package. Sauté mushrooms and onions in margarine until tender. Stir in salt, pepper, flour, and paprika. Then stir in milk slowly, cooking and stirring constantly until thick and smooth. Remove from heat. Stir in light cream. Remove skin and bones from drained salmon (or tuna), then flake. Mix fish with noodles, mushroom mixture, and all but a little of the grated cheese. Pour into casserole, sprinkle remaining grated cheese on top. Bake 20-25 minutes.

****CRAB CASSEROLE

Exchanges per serving: 1 serving = 1 bread, 1 fat, 1/2 fruit, 3 meat.
Calories per serving: 325   Yield: 6 servings

2 cups wild rice mix	1 1/2 teaspoons curry powder
1 onion, chopped fine	2 1/4 cups frozen crab meat
1 stalk celery, chopped fine	1/2 teaspoon monosodium
2 tablespoons salad oil	glutamate (optional)
1 apple, pared and chopped	1/4 cup raisins

Preheat oven to 375°. Cook rice as directed but omit margarine or butter and decrease cooking time to 20 minutes (it will be moist). In a large skillet sauté onion and celery in oil until onion is golden. Stir in apple, curry powder, crab meat (which has been thawed and drained thoroughly), monosodium glutamate, and raisins. Divide mixture into small casserole dishes. Cover and bake 15 minutes.

****FISH OVEN STYLE

Exchanges per serving: 1 serving = 1 fat, 4 meat.
Calories per serving: 337   Yield: 3 servings

1 pound fish steaks (swordfish, halibut, haddock, etc.)
cut into 3 serving pieces

1 tablespoon diet margarine
1/16 teaspoon salt
1/16 teaspoon pepper

Preheat oven to 350°. Remove skin from fish steaks, if necessary, and place without touching one another in the bottom of shallow baking dish. Dot with margarine, then sprinkle salt and pepper on top. Bake until fish flakes with a fork (about 15-20 minutes).

****CRAB (or LOBSTER) AND TOMATOES

Exchanges per serving: 1 serving = 1 1/2 fat, 3 meat, 1/2 milk, 1 "A"
                                    vegetable.
Calories per serving: 350   Yield: 4 servings

4 tomatoes, salted to taste
3 tablespoons onion, chopped fine
3 tablespoons green pepper, chopped fine
2 tablespoons diet margarine
3/4 tablespoon arrowroot powder
1 1/2 cups milk

1 1/2 cups crab (or lobster) meat
1 teaspoon Worcestershire sauce
1/16 teaspoon cayenne pepper
1/2 teaspoon salt
1/2 cup milk cheese, well grated

Preheat oven to 350°. Cut off stem of tomato; cut around inside (be careful not to break shell). Scoop out pulp (this leaves the shell which is about 1/2" thick). Salt to taste, let drain upside down about 10 minutes. Sauté onion and pepper in margarine until onion is golden brown. Mix in arrowroot, stirring constantly. Add milk and heat until this is thick and smooth; then stir in crab (or lobster) meat, Worcestershire sauce, cayenne, and salt. Heat to boil. Fill tomato shells with mixture and garnish with cheese. Place tomatoes in shallow baking pan; add 1/4" water to pan and bake until cheese melts (about 10 minutes). Serve at once.

*SWEET-SOUR TONGUE

Exchanges per serving: 1 slice = 1 meat, 1/4 fat.
Calories per serving: 88   Yield: 4 servings

2 tablespoons diet margarine
1 tablespoon arrowroot powder
1/2 teaspoon salt
1 cup stock

Non-nutritive sweetener
equivalent to 2 tablespoons
sugar
2 tablespoons malt vinegar
1/4 teaspoon pepper

8 slices cooked smoked tongue (3 ounces)

Blend margarine, arrowroot powder, seasonings with stock and cook
until thickened. Add tongue and heat together.

**STUFFED BUNS

Exchanges per serving: 1 bun = 1 bread, 1 1/2 fat, 1 meat.
Calories per serving: 200   Yield: 8 servings

1 6-ounce diet water-packed
tuna (or chicken or turkey)
2 tablespoons green onions,
minced
2 tablespoons celery, minced
1 tablespoon ripe olives,
chopped

Minced dill pickle to taste
1/2 cup diet mayonnaise
1/4 cup cheddar cheese,
grated
8 hot dog buns

Mix all ingredients; fill inside of bun. Wrap in foil. Place in 350° oven
about 10-15 minutes until hot and cheese has melted.

**LIVER A LA BOURGEOISE

Exchanges per serving: 3 ounces = 1 fat, 1 1/2 meat, 1/2 "B" vegetable.
Calories per serving: 187   Yield: 8 servings

1 carrot, shredded
1 onion, minced
1 turnip, diced
1 bay leaf
2 tablespoons diet margarine

1 tablespoon arrowroot powder
2 1/2 pounds liver
2 cups water
1/16 teaspoon seasoned salt

1/16 teaspoon lemon pepper

Brown carrot, onion, and turnip with the bay leaf in margarine. Add
arrowroot powder and blend; then add liver and water. Season, then
simmer 1 1/2 to 1 3/4 hours.

***ONION, LIVER, AND CHEESE

Exchanges per serving: 1 serving = 1/2 fat, 3 meat.
Calories per serving: 239

Yield: 6 servings

1 pound beef liver, quartered
1 tablespoon flour
1/16 teaspoon salt
1/16 teaspoon pepper

1/16 teaspoon garlic salt
2 tablespoons diet margarine
1/2 cup cheddar cheese, grated

1 onion, sliced very thin

Remove the skin and veins from the beef liver and cut liver into 1/2" serving pieces. Sprinkle lightly with flour. Shake off excess and sprinkle salt, pepper and garlic salt on each side. Sauté liver in margarine a few minutes over medium heat. Turn off heat. Pour off most of margarine and return pan to burner; sprinkle pieces with cheese, then thin rounds of onion. Cover. Heat until cheese is melted, then serve.

***FRANKFURTER CASSEROLE

Exchanges per serving: 1 serving = 1 bread, 2 fat, 1 meat, 1 "B" vegetable.

Calories per serving: 260

Yield: 8 servings

1 1/4 cups bean and bacon soup, undiluted
1 1/4 cups water
2 cups all-meat frankfurters, cut into 1/2" slices

1 onion, chopped fine
1 green pepper, chopped fine
1/2 cup celery, chopped fine
2 tablespoons prepared mustard

1 cup ready-mix type biscuits

Preheat oven to 375°. Mix all ingredients except biscuits. Boil gently 5 minutes. Put about 3/4 cup mixture into each of 8 individual baking dishes and top each with biscuit. Bake until biscuits are dark golden brown (about 20 minutes). Serve at once.

**CALIFORNIA POT ROAST

Exchanges per serving: 2 ounces = 2 meat.
Calories per serving: 150

Yield: 20 servings

4 pounds beef rump
2 tablespoons flour
1 teaspoon salt
1/16 teaspoon pepper
1 tablespoon oil
1 onion, chopped fine

2 carrots, sliced
1 tablespoon Worcestershire sauce
1 cup water
Non-nutritive sweetener equivalent to 1/2 cup sugar

Dredge meat well in flour, salt, and pepper. Brown in oil in skillet; add remaining ingredients. Cover. Simmer about 4 hours over low heat.

**ROAST BEEF WITH FRUIT SAUCE

Exchanges per serving: 1 ounce = 1 meat exchange.
1/4 cup sauce = 1 fruit exchange.
Calories per serving: 40 (sauce)   Yield: 3 cups (or 1 dozen 1/4 cups)
75 (meat)

Trim fat from beef before roasting. Salt and pepper. After roasting, trim remaining fat.

Sauce

4 cups artificially sweetened plums (reserve syrup)
1/4 teaspoon salt
1/8 teaspoon pepper
1 tablespoon arrowroot powder

1/3 cup unsweetened frozen orange juice concentrate
2 tablespoons Worcestershire sauce
1/8 teaspoon Tabasco sauce

Drain plums, and pit. Save 3/4 cup of the syrup. Puree plums until smooth; add syrup and balance of ingredients. Blend until smooth. In medium saucepan heat to boiling. Serve over Roast Beef.

***HAMBURGER CORNMEAL SHEPHERD'S PIE

Exchanges per serving: 1 serving = 1/2 bread, 2 fat, 1 1/2 meat, 1/2 "B" vegetable.
Calories per serving: 240
Yield: 8 servings

1/2 cup green pepper, chopped fine
1/4 cup onion, minced fine
2 cups ground round
5 tablespoons oil
1 cup tomato sauce
2 tablespoons catsup
2 teaspoons salt
Dash lemon pepper

1 teaspoon chili powder
1/2 cup flour, sifted
3/4 cup yellow cornmeal
Non-nutritive sweetener equivalent to 1 tablespoon sugar
2 teaspoons baking powder
1/2 teaspoon thyme
1/4 cup (1 medium) egg

1/2 cup skim milk

Preheat oven to 400°. Sauté pepper, onion, beef in 2 tablespoons of oil in skillet, until beef is well browned. Stir in tomato sauce, catsup, 1 teaspoon salt, lemon pepper, and chili powder. Put into 1 1/2-quart casserole. Stir flour, cornmeal, sweetener, baking powder, remaining salt and thyme together in a bowl; then add egg, milk, and rest of oil. Stir until smooth. Top the first mixture with the second and bake, uncovered, until cornbread is slightly brown and firm to touch (about 1/2 hour). Loosen cornbread with a knife around edges, turn on serving plate with top side down.

***MEAT CASSEROLE

Exchanges per serving: 1 4-ounce serving = 1 bread, 3 meat, 1 "A" vegetable.

Calories per serving: 280   Yield: 4 servings

3/4 cup noodles, uncooked
2 1/2 cups tomato juice
2 cups celery, chopped fine
1/2 cup green pepper, chopped fine

2 cups meat, cooked and cubed
1/8 teaspoon pepper
1 1/2 teaspoons salt
1/2 teaspoon diet margarine

Heat oven to 350°. Combine all ingredients. Turn into well-greased casserole; bake 2 hours and 15 minutes.

***SPAGHETTI AND SAUCE

Exchanges per serving: 1 serving = 1 bread, 3 meat, 1 "A" vegetable.
Calories per serving: 285   Yield: 8 servings

3 cups ground round
1 cup onion, chopped fine
1 1/2 cups celery, chopped fine
2 cloves garlic, minced very fine
1/2 cup fresh mushrooms, sliced thin

2 tablespoons oil
3/4 cup tomato paste
1 1/2 cups tomato juice
2 teaspoons salt
1/16 teaspoon pepper
1/4 cup thin spaghetti

Brown meat well; sauté onion, celery, garlic, and mushrooms in oil until onion is golden brown. Add tomato paste, tomato juice, salt, and pepper. Cover. Boil for 1 1/2 hours, gently. After cooling, refrigerate overnight. About 20 minutes before serving, cook spaghetti according to package instructions and thoroughly drain. Measure sauce and add enough water to make a total of 5 cups of sauce. Return sauce to pan, cover and boil gently about 10 minutes. Place 1/2 cup (cooked) spaghetti on plate and top with 2/3 cup meat sauce.

***CHILI CON CARNE

Exchanges per serving: 1 serving = 1 bread, 1/2 fat, 2 meat, 1 "A" vegetable.

Calories per serving: 250   Yield: 8 servings

2 cups ground beef
1 cup onion, chopped fine
1 clove garlic, crushed fine
2 tablespoons chili powder

1 1/4 cups condensed tomato soup, undiluted
2 cups kidney beans
1 tablespoon malt vinegar
1/4 teaspoon salt

Brown beef in hot pan; stir in onion, garlic, and chili powder. Cook, stirring often until onion is tender; add rest of ingredients; bring to boil. Reduce heat and simmer, uncovered, stirring occasionally, about 15 minutes.

***POLLY'S CHILI CON CARNE

Exchanges per serving: 1 serving = 1 bread, 1/2 fat, 2 meat, 1 "A" vegetable.

Calories per serving: 250   Yield: 5 servings

1 cup onion, chopped fine
1/2 cup green pepper, chopped fine
2 cups celery, chopped fine
1 clove garlic, sliced thin
1 tablespoon oil

2 cups ground round
2 cups kidney beans, thoroughly drained
2 cups tomatoes
1 tablespoon chili powder
1/2 teaspoon salt

Sauté onion, pepper, celery, and garlic in salad oil until onion is golden brown. Add beef and cook until well browned. Stir in kidney beans, tomatoes, chili powder, and salt; boil uncovered about 45-50 minutes. Just before serving taste to see if more chili is needed.

***CORNED BEEF DINNER

Exchanges per serving: 3-ounce slice = 1 bread, 1 "A" vegetable, 1 "B" vegetable, 3 meat.

Calories per serving: 300   Yield: 6 servings

1 4-pound corned-beef brisket
Water to cover brisket
6 onions

6 carrots
6 parsnips, scraped
3 potatoes, peeled and halved
1 head cabbage

Cover brisket with cold water in Dutch oven and bring to a boil. Drain. Add water to cover and again bring to boil; reduce heat to low. Cover. Cook until nearly tender (about 3 hours), skimming off as much fat as possible from cooking water. Add vegetables. Cook until vegetables are done (about 10-15 minutes more). Remove fat and vegetables from water; drain vegetables and trim fat from meat.

***MEAT LOAF

Exchanges per serving: 1 serving = 1/2 bread, 3 meat.

Calories per serving: 250   Yield: 6 servings

1/4 cup (1 medium) egg
2 cups ground round
3 slices bread, cubed fine
1/4 cup catsup
1/3 cup onion, chopped fine

2 tablespoons green pepper, chopped fine
1 teaspoon salt
1/2 teaspoon dry mustard
1 tablespoon prepared horse-radish, if desired

Preheat oven to 400°. Mix all ingredients well. Form into a loaf. Place in foil-lined baking pan and bake until done (15-20 minutes).

****MEATBALLS WITH CARAWAY SEEDS

Exchanges per serving: 4 meatballs = 1/2 bread, 4 meat.
Calories per serving: 335   Yield: 4 servings

2 cups ground round
1 onion, minced fine
1/4 cup (1 medium) egg
1 teaspoon lemon peel, grated
   fine
1/4 teaspoon pepper
1/2 teaspoon salt
1 tablespoon dried parsley
   flakes

1 cup raw potato, coarsely
   grated
2 1/2 cups water
4 beef bouillon cubes
1 teaspoon arrowroot powder
1/2 teaspoon caraway seeds
1 tablespoon water

Mix first eight ingredients. Form into sixteen meatballs. Bring water to
boil, and in it dissolve the bouillon; then add meatballs and cover
tightly. Gently boil about 1/2 hour. Remove meatballs from broth and
stir arrowroot and caraway seeds, dissolved in water, into broth until
thick and smooth. Pour a little gravy over meatballs, garnish with
parsley, if desired. (Store remaining gravy in tightly covered jar in
refrigerator for later use.)

****HAMBURGERS

Exchanges per serving: 1 4-ounce pattie = 1 bread, 4 meat.
Calories per serving: 370   Yield: 4 servings

2 cups ground round
1/4 cup (1 medium) egg
1 onion, chopped fine
1 tablespoon horseradish
1 teaspoon salt
1/2 teaspoon pepper

1/2 teaspoon celery seed
1 tablespoon Worcestershire
   sauce
1/2 bun per person, or 1 slice
   bread

Mix all ingredients (except bun) and shape into patties. Broil about 6-7
minutes per side. Serve on bun (or 1 slice bread).

****MEATBALLS

Exchanges per serving: 4 meatballs = 1 bread, 2 meat, 1/2 milk.
Calories per serving: 310   Yield: 6 servings

2 cups ground round
1/4 cup dried bread crumbs
1 teaspoon salt
1 1/2 cups buttermilk
3/4 cup minute rice

1 teaspoon diet margarine
1 cup water
1/2 tablespoon arrowroot
   powder

Mix beef, crumbs, salt, 1/2 cup buttermilk, and rice. Shape into two dozen meatballs (about 1" round). In large skillet brown meatballs in margarine on all sides; pour water over and cover tightly. Boil until rice is tender and meat is cooked (about 30 minutes). Remove from skillet. Mix remaining 1 cup buttermilk with arrowroot to form smooth paste and stir this into liquid remaining in skillet. Stir constantly. Cook until gravy is thick (do not boil). Return meatballs to pan and gently heat. Serve with gravy.

****HEARTY HASH

Exchanges per serving: 1 serving = 1/2 bread, 3 meat, 1/4 skim milk, 1/2 "A" and 1/2 "B" vegetable.

Calories per serving: 325

Yield: 4 servings

1/2 cup onion, ground
1/4 cup parsley, chopped
1 cup cooked potatoes, chopped
2 tablespoons green pepper, ground
1 teaspoon salt

1 1/2 cups leftover cooked beef, diced, chopped, or ground
2 teaspoons Worcestershire sauce
1 tablespoon diet margarine
2/3 cup skim milk (or unsweetened tomato sauce)

Preheat oven to 350°. Mix all ingredients. Pour into a well-greased casserole. Bake about 1/2 hour.

****STUFFED FLANK STEAK

Exchanges per serving: 4 ounces = 1/2 bread, 1 fat, 4 meat.
Calories per serving: 340

Yield: 8 servings

2-pound flank steak
1/16 teaspoon salt
1/16 teaspoon lemon pepper
1 tablespoon flour
4 cups bread cubes
2 small onions, chopped fine

3/4 cup celery, chopped fine
1 1/2 teaspoons sage
1/2 teaspoon Mei Yen seasoning
3 tablespoons diet margarine
1/2 cup water

Preheat oven to 350°. Score steak lightly, crosswise. Sprinkle with salt and pepper and dredge with flour (pound it well into the steak). Combine next five ingredients and spread over steak. Roll meat and tie, or fasten edge with toothpicks. Brown in margarine, then add water; cover and cook about 1 1/2 hours, until tender. Baste occasionally.

****MARGARET'S MEAT PIE

Exchanges per serving: 1 serving = 1 bread, 3 meat, 1/2 milk.
Calories per serving: 325   Yield: 6 servings

1/4 cup onion, chopped fine
1 clove garlic, minced fine
1 tablespoon oil
1 cup oat bread crumbs
1 whole egg plus 2 eggs separated
2 1/4 cups buttermilk
1/4 cup catsup
1 1/2 cups ground meat
2 1/2 teaspoons salt

1/8 teaspoon pepper
1/2 cup yellow cornmeal
1 teaspoon salt
1/2 teaspoon baking soda
Non-nutritive sweetener equivalent to 1 teaspoon sugar
1/4 cup Parmesan cheese, grated

Preheat oven to 350°. Sauté onion and garlic in oil until onion is golden. Remove from heat and stir in oat crumbs, whole egg (1/4 cup), 1/4 cup buttermilk, catsup, meat, 1 1/2 teaspoons salt, and pepper. Line bottom and sides of 10" pie tin with this mixture. Bake 15 minutes: pour off any excess liquid. Mix together rest of buttermilk, cornmeal, remaining salt, baking soda, and sweetener in medium saucepan. Cook, stirring constantly until thick and smooth. Remove from heat. Stir in egg yolks. Beat egg whites until peaks form; fold into cornmeal mix. Fill meat-pie shell. Top with cheese and bake until cheese is lightly brown (about 30 minutes). Let cool for five minutes before serving.

****MISSISSIPPI CASSEROLE

Exchanges per serving: 1 serving = 1/2 bread, 4 meat, 1 fruit.
Calories per serving: 410   Yield: 4 servings

4 large cooked sweet potatoes
2 cups pork sausage
4 large apples, sliced
1/16 teaspoon salt

1/4 cup water
Non-nutritive sweetener equivalent to 1/4 cup brown sugar

Preheat oven to 350°. Peel potatoes. Cut in thin slices. Place half in bottom of greased casserole. Cover with sausage, shaped in 4 cakes. Add apples, sprinkle with salt, then cover with remaining potatoes. Brush with water; sprinkle with sweetener. Bake 1 hour.

***ROAST LEG OF LAMB

Exchanges per serving: 3 ounces = 3 meat.
Calories per serving: 225   Yield: 10-12 servings

5-6 pound leg of lamb   1/8 cup flour
1 clove garlic   1 teaspoon ginger
2-3 teaspoons Bouquet Garni   1 teaspoon seasoned salt
          1 teaspoon lemon pepper

Preheat oven to 300°. Wipe meat with damp cloth. Do not remove the fell — the paperlike covering over the meat. Make gashes in roast with sharp knife; cut garlic into slivers and insert a piece in each gash. Rub meat with condiments and dredge with flour. Place, fat side up and uncovered, in shallow roaster. Roast until tender (about 30-35 minutes per pound). Remove garlic and serve.

****VEAL A LA KING

Exchanges per serving: 3 ounces = 1/2 bread, 4 meat, 1/4 skim milk.
Calories per serving: 346   Yield: 16 servings

1/2 cup green pepper, chop-   4 cups skim milk
   ped fine   1/16 teaspoon seasoned salt
1/2 cup mushrooms   1/16 teaspoon pepper
3 tablespoons diet margarine   4 cups cooked veal, diced
3 tablespoons arrowroot pow-   1 pimiento, diced
   der   8 slices toast

Cook pepper and mushrooms in margarine for 8 minutes; remove vegetables. Add arrowroot to margarine and blend. Add skim milk and seasonings and cook until thickened, stirring constantly. Add green pepper, mushrooms, veal, and pimiento and heat. Serve on one-half slice toast.

**SAUERKRAUT AND SPARERIBS

Exchanges per serving: 2 ounces = 2 meat.
Calories per serving: 150   Yield: 6 servings

1 quart sauerkraut   4 pounds spareribs
Non-nutritive sweetener   1/16 teaspoon seasoned salt
   equivalent to 1/4 cup brown   1/16 teaspoon pepper
   sugar   1/2 cup hot water

Preheat oven to 350°. Place sauerkraut in greased baking dish. Sprinkle with sweetener. Brown spareribs under broiler. Season, place on sauerkraut, and add hot water. Cover. Bake 45 minutes to 1 hour.

**HAM LOAF

Exchanges per serving: 1 serving = 1/2 bread, 2 meat.
Calories per serving: 200   Yield: 16 servings

1 1/2 pounds ham, ground well
1 pound beef, ground well
1/2 cup (2 medium) eggs, beaten
1 1/4 cups milk
4 slices soft bread, broken into small pieces
1 1/2 teaspoons salt

Dash pepper
Non-nutritive sweetener equivalent to 3/4 cup sugar
1/4 teaspoon cinnamon
1/4 teaspoon cloves
1/4 teaspoon nutmeg
1/2 teaspoon dry mustard
1/2 teaspoon vegetable oil

Preheat oven to 350°. Combine all ingredients except oil and mix well. Use oil to grease loaf pan and place mix in pan. Bake 1 1/2 hours.

***BAKED HAM OR HAM STEAK WITH PINEAPPLE

Exchanges per servings: 3 ounces = 1 fruit, 3 meat.
Calories per serving: 260   Yield: 24 servings

1 6-8 pound canned ham
Non-nutritive sweetener equivalent to 1/2 cup sugar
1 teaspoon dry mustard

1/2 cup bread crumbs
3/4 cup pineapple juice
5-6 slices unsweetened pineapple

Preheat oven to 300°. Spread ham with mixture of sweetener, mustard, and bread crumbs. Add pineapple juice. Bake 15 minutes then add slices of pineapple and cook entire dish an additional 45 minutes.

****HAWAIIAN BAKED PORK

Exchanges per serving: 1 serving = 1 bread, 1 fat, 1/2 fruit, 3 meat.
Calories per serving: 344   Yield: 4 servings

2 cups crushed unsweetened pineapple
3 medium-sized sweet potatoes
Non-nutritive sweetener equivalent to 3 3/4 cups brown sugar

4 shoulder pork steaks (3 ounces each)
1/16 teaspoon salt
1/16 teaspoon pepper
4 bacon strips

Preheat oven to 350°. Place pineapple in one large baking dish, or in 4 individual ones. Pare and slice sweet potatoes and place these over pineapple. Sprinkle with sweetener. Season pork steaks with salt and pepper; place these on top of sweet potatoes; then arrange bacon strips on top of pork steaks. Cover and bake 1 hour, or until tender. Remove cover; increase temperature to 450° for the last 10 minutes to brown steak and bacon.

***PORK ROAST WITH SPICE SAUCE

Exchanges per serving: 3 ounces = 3 meat.
Calories per serving: 219

Yield: 12 servings

1 4-5 pound fresh picnic shoulder of pork
1/16 teaspoon salt
1/16 teaspoon pepper
2 small onions, minced
1 tablespoon Worcestershire sauce

Non-nutritive sweetener equivalent to 1 1/2 cups sugar
1/2 teaspoon paprika
1/2 cup vinegar
1/2 cup water
2 tablespoons catsup

Have butcher bone and roll roast. Salt, pepper, and place fat side up on rack in open roaster. Roast at 350° for 40-45 minutes per pound. Combine the other ingredients and cook together for 5 minutes. Pour over roast and serve.

***PORK PATTIES IN GRAVY

Exchanges per serving: 1 serving = 1/2 bread, 1/2 fat, 2 meat, 1 "B" vegetable.
Calories per serving: 220

Yield: 8 servings

2 cups very lean pork shoulder, ground
1/2 cup (2 medium) eggs
1/2 cup skim milk
4 slices dry bread, cubed fine
9 onions, one chopped fine, rest only peeled
1 1/2 teaspoons salt

1/3 teaspoon pepper
3/4 teaspoon nutmeg
2 tablespoons salad oil
1/2 cup water
1 1/4 cups undiluted, condensed beef bouillon
1 teaspoon oregano
1/4 teaspoon paprika

Mix first eight ingredients well and let stand a few minutes. Then divide into patties. Brown these well in oil on both sides; then drain on brown paper or paper towel. Pour fat from pan and add the rest of ingredients. Return patties to mixture, cover, cook gently 1/2 hour.

***MAINE SUPPER

Exchanges per serving: 1 cup = 2 1/2 bread, 1/2 fat, 1 1/4 meat.
Calories per serving: 281

Yield: 6 cups

1 tablespoon onion, chopped
2 tablespoons green pepper, chopped
2 tablespoons diet margarine
4 cups pork and beans

Non-nutritive sweetener equivalent to 1 1/2 cups brown sugar
1/2 cup chopped celery
1 cup Vienna sausage, sliced in half

Brown onion and pepper in margarine. Add pork and beans, sweetener, and celery. Mix together and place in individual casseroles. Place 3 sausages in each casserole and bake at 350° until browned.

***CHICKEN LIVERS

Exchanges per serving: 1 serving = 1 fat, 3 meat, 1 "A" and 1 "B" vegetable.

Calories per serving: 279   Yield: 4 servings

2 onions, sliced thin
2 stalks celery, sliced thin
1 tablespoon diet margarine
1 pound chicken livers
1/2 teaspoon salt
1/2 teaspoon pepper

Sauté onions and celery in margarine until celery is wilted. Remove and place to one side. Add chicken livers and turn heat high; cook, turning once or twice until done (3-5 minutes). Top with onions and celery. Season with salt and pepper.

***CHARLOTTE'S CURRIED CHICKEN

Exchanges per serving: 1/2 cup sauce over 1/2 cup rice = 1 bread, 1/4 fruit, 2 meat.

Calories per serving: 224   Yield: 6 servings

1 cup long-grain white rice
2 chicken breasts, split, boned, and cut into 2" or 3" pieces
1 cup mushrooms, sliced thin
1/3 cup onions, chopped fine
1 tablespoon diet margarine
1 chicken bouillon cube
1 teaspoon salt
1 1/2 teaspoons curry powder
1/2 tablespoon arrowroot powder
3/4 cup skim milk
1 cup water
1 cup apples, sliced
1 teaspoon parsley, chopped fine

Cook rice as directed, but omit margarine. Sauté chicken, mushrooms, and onions in margarine until chicken is lightly browned on all sides (about 15 minutes). Make a smooth paste of bouillon cube, salt, curry powder, and arrowroot; then add milk, water, apple, and parsley. Cook until thick and smooth and apple is tender, stirring constantly. Stir chicken into sauce and pour onto the rice.

***CHICKEN SUPERB

Exchanges per serving: 1 serving = 1 fat, 1/4 fruit, 3 meat.
Calories per serving: 274   Yield: 4 servings

1/4 cup flour
1 1/16 teaspoons salt
1/8 teaspoon pepper
2 chicken breasts, split and skinned
2 tablespoons diet margarine
1/2 green pepper, chopped fine
1/4 cup pimiento, diced fine
1/2 cup mushrooms, cut in quarters
1/4 teaspoon ginger
1 cup canned chicken broth
1/4 cup orange juice
1/2 orange, unpeeled and sliced thin

Mix together flour, 1 teaspoon salt, half the pepper. Lightly coat chicken. Cook chicken in margarine until golden, using a tightly covered pan. Then turn breasts, meat side down, and add rest of ingredients. Cover. Stir occasionally while boiling gently, until tender (about 1/2 hour).

****BROILED SPRING CHICKEN

Exchanges per serving: 4 ounces = 4 meat.
Calories per serving: 300   Yield: 16 servings

1 4-pound broiling chicken, dressed
2 tablespoons diet margarine, melted
1/16 teaspoon seasoned salt
1/16 teaspoon lemon pepper

Preheat oven to 500°. Wash chicken inside and out. Brush with margarine. Rub with salt and pepper. Place in broiler; brown evenly, turn and brown other side. Allow 30 minutes or more to cook so the joints are not rare. Baste from time to time, adding water if needed.

****CHICKEN DELIGHT

Exchanges per serving: 1 serving = 1 bread, 1 1/2 fat, 3 meat, 1 "A", 1 "B" vegetable.
Calories per serving: 398   Yield: 5 servings

2 pounds chicken breasts, boned and split
1 cup long-grain rice
3 tablespoons oil
1 green pepper, chopped fine
3 stalks celery, cut in 2" pieces
1 small onion, chopped fine
1 chicken bouillon cube
1/2 cup water chestnuts, drained and sliced thin
1 teaspoon salt
1/4 teaspoon ginger
3/4 cup water
1 teaspoon arrowroot powder
1 tablespoon soy sauce
1-pound can bean sprouts, drained thoroughly

Remove any fat or gristle from chicken, split each piece into two thin layers, then cut layers into strips about 2" long and 1/4" wide. Cook rice according to directions on the package (omit margarine). Heat oil in skillet; add chicken. Cook, covered, over high heat. Stir constantly until chicken turns completely white and is slightly browned (about 2 minutes). Turn heat to medium and add green pepper, celery, onion, bouillon cube, water chestnuts, salt, ginger, and water. Make a smooth paste of arrowroot and soy sauce and stir this into chicken mixture until smooth. Boil gently 6-7 minutes, tightly covered. Add bean sprouts to cooked vegetables; cover and boil gently another 2 minutes. Each serving consists of 1/2 cup cooked rice with 1 cup chicken mixture.

SAUCES

Notes

GRAVIES AND APPROXIMATE EXCHANGES

Arrowroot: 1 tablespoon = 1 slice bread. (May be used for fruit juices.)

Cornstarch: 2 tablespoons = 1 slice bread. (May be used for fruit juices.)

Egg Yolk: Used in place of 1 tablespoon flour = 1 fat exchange. (Yields 3 grams protein and 5 fat, no carbohydrate. *N. B.* This is of different food value than flour.)

Flour: 1 tablespoon = 1/3 bread exchange.
3 tablespoons = 1 bread exchange.
(Use all-purpose flour and sift.)

Tapioca: 1 teaspoon = None. (Use mostly for sweet sauces. In thickening power this is equivalent to 1 tablespoon flour.)

Nondairy whipping cream may be Dream Whip, Cool Whip, etc., any of your choice.
Imitation sour cream may be Imo, etc., any of your choice.
Granulated sweeteners are preferred for recipes for solids such as cake. Liquid sweeteners may be used for such things as drinks.

SUBSTITUTE SUGAR SYRUPS AND GLAZES

Consult notes on Special Ingredients.

*BERRY SAUCE

Exchanges per serving: 1 tablespoon = None.
Calories per serving: 0   Yield: 1 1/2 cups

Non-nutritive sweetener equivalent to 1/2 cup sugar
1 teaspoon arrowroot powder
1/16 teaspoon salt
1/2 cup water

1 cup berries (blueberries, raspberries, etc.)
1 tablespoon lemon juice
1 teaspoon lemon rind, grated

Combine sweetener, arrowroot, and salt, then stir in water and add berries. Bring to a boil, simmer until clear and thick, about 5 minutes. Remove from heat and add lemon juice and rind. Chill and use over ice creams, custards, plain cakes, waffles, or pancakes.

*BARB'S BARBECUE SAUCE

Exchanges per serving: 1/2 cup = 1/4 "A" and 1/4 "B" vegetable.
Calories per serving: 0   Yield: 2 cups

1/2 cup onions, chopped fine
2/3 cup tomato paste
1 cup water
1 teaspoon Worcestershire sauce
2 cups dietetic maple topping
2 tablespoons garlic-flavored vinegar

1/4 cup catsup (see next recipe)
1 teaspoon salt
1/8 teaspoon pepper
1/4 teaspoon dried oregano, crushed fine
1/4 teaspoon dried rosemary, crushed fine

Blend all ingredients together in a saucepan. Simmer over low heat about half an hour, or until onions are well cooked. Use with any broiled meat such as lamb patties, ground beef, beef, pork, or lamb chops.

*CATSUP

Exchanges per serving: 1 tablespoon = None.
Calories per serving: 0   Yield: 2 cups

4 tomatoes, quartered
1/3 cup green pepper, chopped fine
1/4 cup onions, chopped fine
1/8 cup red pepper, chopped very fine
1/2 cup malt vinegar
1/2 teaspoon salt
Non-nutritive sweetener equivalent to 1 cup sugar

1/4 teaspoon cinnamon
1/8 teaspoon allspice
1/8 teaspoon anise seed, crushed fine
1/4 teaspoon ground mustard
1/4 teaspoon powdered red pepper
1/4 teaspoon mace

If using blender, fill 3/4 full with first four ingredients and blend about 3-4 seconds at highest speed. If not using blender, mix until smoothness of a puree. Pour mixture into pan, adding vinegar, salt, and sweetener. Tie the spices loosely together in a bag of light cheesecloth and add. Simmer, uncovered, until only about 1/2 mixture remains. Remove bag of spices.

*MINT SAUCE

Exchanges per serving: 1 tablespoon = None.
Calories per serving: 0   Yield: 1 3/4 cups

1/4 cup vinegar
1 cup water
1/2 cup mint leaves, chopped
1/4 cup lemon juice

Non-nutritive sweetener equivalent to 1 1/2 tablespoons sugar
1/2 teaspoon salt

Heat vinegar and 1/2 cup water to boiling. Pour over half the mint leaves. Let stand 15 minutes. Strain. Add remaining water, lemon juice, sweetener, and salt. Chill. Add remaining mint leaves. Serve with lamb.

*SWEET AND TANGY TOMATO SAUCE FOR SPARERIBS AND LOIN OF PORK

Exchanges per serving: 1/2 cup = None.
Calories per serving: 0   Serves: 2 1/2 cups

1/3 cup vinegar
Non-nutritive sweetener
  equivalent to 1 1/2 cups
  sugar
2 tablespoons Worcestershire
  sauce

2 tablespoons prepared mustard
1/2 teaspoon Tabasco sauce
1/4 cup minced onion
2 cups tomato sauce

Combine all ingredients in a saucepan, bring to a boil. Use to baste spareribs or loin of pork.

*GRAVY

Exchanges per serving: 1 tablespoon = None.
Calories per serving: 8   Yield: 2 cups

1 onion, thinly sliced
2 stalks celery, diced
1 1/4 cups chicken broth (or
  condensed beef consommé)

1 1/4 cups water
1/4 teaspoon Gravy Master
1 tablespoon arrowroot powder

Combine onion, celery, broth, and water in a medium saucepan; cover and boil gently over low heat until onion is transparent. Strain. Reserve vegetables for later use. Return broth to pan. Use a little water, Gravy Master, and arrowroot to make smooth paste. Stir slowly into broth and heat to boiling.

*HOT SHOYU (SOY) SAUCE

Exchanges per serving: 1 ounce = None.
Calories per serving: 8   Yield: 1 2/3 cups

1 cup soy sauce
2/3 cup water
Non-nutritive sweetener
  equivalent to 1/2 cup brown
  sugar

1/4 teaspoon instant onion
1 teaspoon arrowroot powder

Blend all ingredients and heat to light boil. Serve as dip for Shrimp Tempura, "pupus," or as sauce for fish or chicken.

*BARBECUE SAUCE

Exchanges per serving: 1 tablespoon = None.
Calories per serving: 10   Yield: 2 cups

4 tablespoons lemon juice
1/16 teaspoon red pepper
2 tablespoons cider vinegar
1 cup catsup (see catsup recipe)
1/2 cup water

3 tablespoons Worcestershire sauce
1/16 teaspoon lemon pepper
1 1/2 teaspoons mustard
Non-nutritive sweetener equivalent to 1/2 cup sugar
1/2 teaspoon salt

Combine all ingredients and simmer over medium heat about 20-25 minutes.

*COLD SHOYU (SOY) SAUCE

Exchanges per serving: 1 tablespoon = None.
Calories per serving: 0   Serves: 3/4 cup

1/2 cup soy sauce
Non-nutritive sweetener equivalent to 3 tablespoons brown sugar

2 tablespoons wine vinegar

Blend ingredients well. Serve in small bowls with hot fried foods, or cold meat, or fish "pupus."

*TOMATO SAUCE

Exchanges per serving: 1/4 cup = None.
Calories per serving: 10   Yield: 3 cups

1/2 onion, chopped fine
1 tablespoon olive oil
1/2 clove garlic, minced fine
2 cups tomato sauce
1 cup water

1/4 teaspoon oregano
1/4 teaspoon basil
Non-nutritive sweetener equivalent to 1/4 teaspoon sugar
1/4 teaspoon salt

Sauté onion in oil until lightly browned; add garlic and sauté this until lightly browned also. Stir in sauce, water, and condiments. Simmer 1 hour; if using for spaghetti, simmer 5 hours.

*GOLDEN SHOYU DIP

Exchanges per serving: 1 ounce = 1/4 fat.
Calories per serving: 12   Yield: 1 1/4 cups

1 cup safflower mayonnaise
1/4 cup soy sauce

1/2 teaspoon instant onion
1/4 teaspoon arrowroot powder

Blend all ingredients until smooth. Chill and restir before serving as dip for all fish "pupus" or with grilled or fried fish.

*SWEET AND SOUR MARINADE
For Shish Kabobs and Brochettes

Exchanges per serving: 1/2 cup = None.
Calories per serving: 0

Yield: 2 cups

1 cup soy sauce
1/2 cup vinegar
1/2 cup unsweetened pine-
apple juice

Non-nutritive sweetener equivalent to 1 1/2 cups sugar
1/2 teaspoon salt
1/2 teaspoon garlic powder

Combine all ingredients and bring to a boil. Marinate beef or lamb cubes in mixture for at least four hours. Also useful for basting meat while cooking.

*TANGY TONGUE SAUCE

(Not for diabetics without consent of doctor.)

Exchanges per serving: 1/4 cup = 1/2 fat, 1/2 fruit.
Calories per serving: 43 + alcohol content
(about 90)

Yield: 3 1/4 cups

1/4 cup diet margarine
1/8 cup arrowroot powder
1 1/2 cups unsweetened apple juice
3/4 cup beer

2 tablespoons white vinegar
Non-nutritive sweetener equivalent to 2 tablespoons brown sugar
1/2 cup raisins

Melt margarine, stir in arrowroot powder; gradually add apple juice and beer, stirring constantly. Add rest of the ingredients and cook over low heat, stirring until sauce is smooth and slightly thickened. Serve over hot or cold tongue.

*RAISIN SAUCE

Exchanges per serving: 1 tablespoon = None.
Calories per serving: 16

Yield: 1 1/2 cups

Non-nutritive sweetener equivalent to 3/4 cup brown sugar
1 1/2 tablespoons arrowroot powder

1 1/2 cups broth (preferably tongue)
1 tablespoon fat
1/4 cup vinegar
1/2 cup golden raisins
1 lemon, sliced thin

Mix sweetener and arrowroot powder in top of double boiler. Add broth gradually, stirring constantly. Add remaining ingredients. Cook until raisins are plump and mixture thick. Stir occasionally. Serve hot with ham or tongue.

*TARTAR SAUCE

Exchanges per serving: 2 tablespoons = 1/2 fat.
Calories per serving: 20   Yield: 1/2 cup

1/4 cup dietetic whipped dressing

2 tablespoons dill pickle, chopped

2 tablespoons parsley, minced

1 teaspoon lemon juice

1/4 teaspoon salt

Mix all ingredients together. Chill before serving. Store in refrigerator.

*CELERY AND TOMATO SAUCE

Exchanges per serving: 1/2 cup = 1/2 fat, 1 "A" vegetable
Calories per serving: 23   Yield: 2 cups

1 tablespoon green pepper, minced fine

2 tablespoons dried onion

1 cup celery, sliced thin

1 tablespoon diet margarine

1 scant cup tomato sauce

1/2 teaspoon sesame seeds, crushed fine

1/4 teaspoon lemon pepper

1/16 teaspoon salt

1/16 teaspoon black pepper

1/4 teaspoon garlic salt

Sauté pepper, onion, and celery in margarine until golden and wilted. Add balance of ingredients. Boil gently about half an hour.

*SPAGHETTI SAUCE

Exchanges per serving: 1 cup = 1/3 fat.
Calories per serving: 25   Yield: 10 cups

1/2 cup celery, chopped fine

1 1/2 cups onion, chopped fine

1/4 cup diet margarine

8 cups tomatoes

1 cup tomato sauce

1/2 teaspoon thyme

1/2 teaspoon marjoram

1/8 teaspoon celery salt

1/16 teaspoon garlic salt

1/4 teaspoon rosemary

1 teaspoon oregano

1/2 teaspoon basil

1/4 teaspoon salt

1/16 teaspoon pepper

Sauté celery, and onion in margarine until golden and wilted. Add remaining ingredients. Cover and bring to boil; uncover and boil gently until sauce is thick. Use for noodles, spaghetti, macaroni, or meat. This calorie count does not include calories for spaghetti, noodles, macaroni, or any complementary main course.

*CHINESE MUSTARD

(Not for diabetics without consent of doctor.)

Exchanges per serving: 1 ounce = 1/4 fat.
Calories per serving: 15 + calories for beer or wine   Yield: 1/2 cup

1/3 cup dry mustard
1 tablespoon safflower oil
Non-nutritive sweetener
equivalent to 1 teaspoon
sugar

1/2 teaspoon seasoned salt
2 teaspoons flat beer or wine

Mix all ingredients until smooth; serve in small dipping bowl.

*APPLE CRANBERRY RELISH

Exchanges per serving: 1/4 cup = 1 fat, 1 fruit.
Calories per serving: 85   Yield: 1 3/4 cups

1/2 cup apples, diced
2 cups fresh cranberries,
chopped fine
1/4 cup white raisins, chopped
fine

1/4 cup walnuts, chopped fine
Non-nutritive sweetener
equivalent to 1 cup sugar
1/2 teaspoon lemon juice

Combine all ingredients, mixing well. Chill overnight in refrigerator.

*LOW-CALORIE TOPPING WHIP

Exchanges per serving: 1/4 cup = 1/4 skim milk.
Calories per serving: 16   Yield: 3 1/2 cups

1/2 cup nonfat dry milk
1/2 cup ice water
2 tablespoons fresh lemon
juice

Non-nutritive sweetener
equivalent to 1/4 cup sugar

Place bowl and egg beater in refrigerator for about two hours. Mix
nonfat milk and ice water in chilled bowl, beat with mixer until soft
peaks form. Add juice and sweetener and beat again until mixture
forms stiff peaks.

*CUSTARD SAUCE FOR SHORTCAKES

Exchanges per serving: 1 tablespoon = trace milk.
Calories per serving: 10   Yield: 2 1/2 cups

2 cups skim milk
1/2 cup (2 medium) eggs
Non-nutritive sweetener
equivalent to 1 1/2 cups
sugar

1/2 tablespoon arrowroot
powder
1/4 teaspoon salt
1 teaspoon vanilla extract
1 teaspoon almond extract

Scald milk in saucepan. Beat egg, sweetener, arrowroot, and salt in
small bowl; gradually add in scalded milk. Return mixture to saucepan.
Cook over low heat, stirring constantly until mixture coats a spoon and
is slightly thickened. Remove from heat and beat in vanilla and almond
extracts. Chill until ready to use.

*CHERRY GLAZE

Exchanges per serving: 1/2 cup = 1 fruit.
Calories per serving: 40　　　　　　　　　　　Yield: 3 cups

2 cups sour red cherries, wa-
　ter-packed and pitted
1/2 cup liquid from cherries
Non-nutritive sweetener
　equivalent to 2 tablespoons
　sugar

1 teaspoon arrowroot powder
1 tablespoon lemon juice
1/4 teaspoon almond extract
Drop of red vegetable food
　coloring (optional)

Mix liquid from cherries with sweetener and arrowroot and stir to make
smooth paste. Cook, stirring constantly until thick and smooth. Add
cherries, lemon juice and almond extract. Allow to cool at room
temperature. May be used over dietetic ice cream, pineapple cheese pie,
among other desserts.

*LEMON SAUCE

Exchanges per serving: 1/4 cup = 1 fat.
Calories per serving: 50　　　　　　　　　　　Yield: 1 cup

3/4 tablespoon arrowroot
　powder
Non-nutritive sweetener
　equivalent to 1/2 cup sugar
1/8 teaspoon salt
1 cup boiling water
2 tablespoons diet margarine
1 1/2 tablespoons lemon juice

1 1/2 teaspoons lemon rind,
　ground fine
1/16 teaspoon anise seed,
　crushed fine
1/16 teaspoon nutmeg
1/16 teaspoon cloves, ground
　fine

Combine arrowroot, sweetener, and salt in saucepan; add boiling water
slowly, stirring to avoid lumps. Simmer and stir until thick; remove
from heat. Stir in margarine and remaining ingredients. Use for cake
fillings and over bread puddings and custards.

*CUSTARD SAUCE

Exchanges per serving: 1/2 cup = 3/4 meat, 1/3 skim milk.
Calories per serving: 80　　　　　　　　　　　Yield: 4 servings

1 whole egg plus 2 egg yolks
Non-nutritive sweetener
　equivalent to 3 tablespoons
　sugar

1/8 teaspoon salt
1 1/2 cups skim milk
1 teaspoon vanilla extract

Beat 1 egg and 2 yolks together in saucepan, reserving 2 whites, covered
in refrigerator for use another time. Blend in sweetener and salt and
gradually stir in skim milk. Place over low heat, stirring constantly
until mixture slightly thickens and coats a metal spoon. Remove from
heat. Stir in vanilla. Chill. (Sauce will thicken during chilling.)

*POLLY'S CUSTARD SAUCE

Exchanges per serving: 1/2 cup = 1/2 meat, 1/2 skim milk.
Calories per serving: 75

Yield: 3 1/2 cups

3 cups skim milk
Non-nutritive sweetener
equivalent to 1/2 cup sugar
1 teaspoon almond extract

1 tablespoon arrowroot powder
1/2 cup (3 medium) egg yolks

Combine skim milk and sweetener in top of double boiler and heat. Mix arrowroot powder and egg yolks and beat well. Add small amount of hot milk mixture to egg mixture and blend. Return entire mixture to top of double boiler and cook over simmering water. Stir constantly (about 15 minutes) until mixture is slightly thickened. Remove from heat at once; pour into Pyrex bowl. Stir in almond extract and place in refrigerator to chill. It will thicken as it chills.

*ORANGE SAUCE

Exchanges per serving: 1/4 cup = 1 fruit.
Calories per serving: 40

Yield: 2 cups

Non-nutritive sweetener
equivalent to 1 cup sugar
1/4 teaspoon salt
1 tablespoon arrowroot powder
1 teaspoon grated lemon peel

1 cup orange juice
1/4 cup lemon juice
3/4 cup boiling water
1 tablespoon diet margarine
1 teaspoon grated orange peel

Combine sweetener, salt, and arrowroot. Stir in orange and lemon juices, and boiling water. Boil 1 minute, stirring constantly. Remove from heat and stir in margarine, orange and lemon peels. Serve over hot cake or pudding.

*SAUCE ROYALE

Exchanges per serving: 1/2 cup = 1 fat.
Calories per serving: 52

Yield: 4 servings

1 tablespoon arrowroot powder
1/2 teaspoon nutmeg
1/2 teaspoon cinnamon
1/8 teaspoon allspice
2 tablespoons diet margarine

4 tablespoons cold water
2 cups boiling water
1/16 teaspoon salt
Non-nutritive sweetener
equivalent to 1 cup sugar

Dissolve arrowroot and spices in cold water; add to boiling water. Stir, bring to simmer, then add salt, sweetener, and margarine. Use hot for custards.

*CITRUS FRUIT SAUCE

Exchanges per servings: 1/4 cup = 3/4 fat.
Calories per serving: 40   Yield: 1 cup

Non-nutritive sweetener
  equivalent to 1/2 cup sugar
3/4 tablespoon arrowroot
  powder
1/8 teaspoon salt
1 cup boiling water
2 tablespoons diet margarine,
  melted

1 1/2 tablespoons fruit juice
  (grapefruit, lemon, or orange)
1 1/2 teaspoons grated fruit
  rind
1/16 teaspoon nutmeg

Combine sweetener, arrowroot, and salt in a saucepan. Stir in boiling
water until smooth; stir and simmer until clear and thick; stir in balance
of ingredients.

*SAUCE CHERRIE

Exchanges per serving: 1/2 cup = 1 fruit.
Calories per serving: 40   Yield: 2 cups

1 teaspoon arrowroot powder
2 cups water-packed cherries
1/2 teaspoon almond extract

1/2 teaspoon vanilla extract
Non-nutritive sweetener
  equivalent to 1/2 cup sugar

Combine arrowroot and cherries; bring to boil and simmer 5-6 minutes.
Remove from heat and add extracts and sweetener. Serve when slightly
warm. Can be used over dietetic ice cream, custards, and the like.

*CREAM SAUCE

Exchanges per serving: 1/2 cup = 1/4 milk.
Calories per serving: 45   Yield: 2 1/4 cups

4 tablespoons instant dry milk
  powder
1 tablespoon arrowroot powder

1/8 teaspoon lemon pepper
1/2 teaspoon seasoned salt
2 cups water

If using blender, blend all ingredients until completely blended; if not
using blender, mix to puree smoothness. Cook over low heat.

**CHOCOLATE SAUCE

Exchanges per serving: 1 tablespoon = 2 1/2 fat.
Calories per serving: 105   Yield: 1 cup

1 cup unsweetened chocolate, shaved
1/4 cup water

Non-nutritive sweetener equivalent to 1/4 cup sugar
1/2 cup cream

Combine chocolate, water, and sweetener. Melt over hot water in double boiler. Stir until smooth, remove from heat, and blend in cream. Serve either hot or cold.

**MAPLE-FLAVORED SAUCE

Exchanges per serving: 1/4 cup = 1 fat, 1/2 milk.
Calories per serving: 130   Yield: 1 3/4 cups

1/4 cup diet margarine
1 tablespoon arrowroot powder
Non-nutritive sweetener equivalent to 1 cup sugar

1/2 cup water
1 cup evaporated milk
1 1/2 teaspoons maple flavoring

Melt margarine. Blend in arrowroot powder; add sweetener, water, and milk. Cook over medium heat, stirring constantly until thick; remove from heat. Add maple flavoring and chill.

**HAWAIIAN CURRY SAUCE

Exchanges per serving: 1/2 cup = 1 fat, 1/2 fruit, 1/2 skim milk.
Calories per serving: 105   Yield: 2 cups

1/4 cup safflower oil
1 onion, minced
2 apples, peeled and diced
2 1/2 teaspoons arrowroot powder
2 cups coconut milk or skim milk

1 teaspoon garlic salt
1 teaspoon salt
1 teaspoon ground ginger
3 tablespoons soy sauce
1 to 3 teaspoons curry powder

Heat oil. Add onion and apples. Cover and cook 10 minutes, stirring occasionally. Add arrowroot and stir until smooth; add coconut or skim milk with garlic salt, salt, ginger, soy sauce, and curry powder, stirring constantly until mixture thickens and boils. Reduce heat to very low, cover and cook 20 minutes. Mix sauce with 2 cups cooked seafood, chicken, or meat and serve on steamed rice, or as called for in recipe.

VEGETABLES

PROXIMATE COMPOSITION OF
CAMPBELL SOUP COMPANY PRODUCTS

(Contents of 100 grams, equivalent to one 3 1/2-ounce can. This makes one serving when prepared according to the directions.)

	Cal- ories	Pro- tein gm	Fat gm	Car- bohy- drate gm	So- dium mg	Vita- min A I. U.
JUICES						
Campbell's Tomato						
Juice	20	0.8	0.1	4.0	365	620
"V-8" Cocktail						
Vegetable Juice	19	0.8	0.1	3.6	365	1260

*EGGPLANT, PEPPER, AND MUSHROOMS

Exchanges per serving: 1 cup = 1/2 fat, 1 "A" vegetable.
Calories per serving: 23   Yield: 12 cups

1 large eggplant, cut and diced into squares
1/3 cup oil
1/2 cup water
2 large green peppers, cut and diced
1 cup sliced mushrooms, drained
2 cups tomatoes, peeled and diced
1 clove garlic, minced very fine
1 teaspoon salt
Non-nutritive sweetener equivalent to 1 teaspoon sugar
1/2 teaspoon pepper

Place the squares of eggplant (unpeeled) into frying pan in which 3 tablespoons of oil have been heated. Sauté over medium heat 2 minutes, turning often. Add 2 tablespoons water. Cover and cook, adding water, 2 tablespoons at a time as it is absorbed. Turn eggplant until tender (about 10 minutes). Remove eggplant from pan into a bowl; add balance of oil to pan and sauté peppers about 10 minutes; heat mushrooms until soft. Add these to eggplant. Place tomato, garlic, salt, sweetener, and pepper in a pan. Simmer until it makes a thick sauce and pour over eggplant. Mix lightly.

*EGGPLANT DELIGHT

Exchanges per serving: 1 cup = 1/2 fat, 1 "A" and 1 "B" vegetable.
Calories per serving: 60   Yield: 6 cups

1 onion, sliced thin	3 cups eggplant, peeled, sliced,
1/4 green pepper, chopped fine	and cubed
	2 cups tomatoes
2 tablespoons diet margarine	1/2 teaspoon salt

1/8 teaspoon pepper

Sauté onion and pepper in margarine until soft, in medium skillet, tightly covered. Add eggplant cubes, tomatoes, salt and pepper, and cover. Boil until eggplant is tender (about 10 minutes).

*DORIS' CREAMED MUSHROOMS

Exchanges per serving: 1/2 cup = 1 fat, 1 "B" vegetable.
Calories per serving: 80   Yield: 6 cups

1 envelope dry cream of mushroom soup mix	3 tablespoons diet margarine
	1 tablespoon lemon juice
2 cups water	1/16 teaspoon salt
4 cups fresh mushrooms	1/16 teaspoon pepper

Add soup mix to water, gently boil, stirring now and then, for about 10 minutes. In a large skillet sauté mushrooms in margarine until browned on all sides. Pour soup and lemon juice over mushrooms. Season.

*CREAMED SPINACH

Exchanges per serving: 2/3 cup = 1/2 fat, 1 "A" vegetable.
Calories per serving: 40   Yield: 2 cups

1 clove garlic, minced fine	1/2 teaspoon salt
1 tablespoon diet margarine	1/8 teaspoon pepper
1 1/4 cups frozen spinach, chopped	1/2 tablespoon arrowroot powder

1/2 cup milk

Sauté garlic in margarine until brown, then discard garlic. Add spinach, which has been thawed thoroughly, salt, and pepper. Cover tightly and separate with fork occasionally. Cook over low heat until spinach is tender and all liquid evaporated (about 4-5 minutes). Form a smooth, thin paste of arrowroot powder and milk and add to cooked spinach. Heat, stirring constantly until thick and smooth.

*GOURMET SPINACH

Exchanges per serving: 1 serving = 1 fat, 1 "B" vegetable.
Calories per serving: 80   Yield: 6 servings

1 cup mushrooms, sliced thin	1 1/4 cups frozen spinach,
1 onion, chopped fine	chopped
1 clove garlic, minced	1/3 cup imitation sour cream
1 tablespoon diet margarine	1 1/16 teaspoons salt
	1/8 teaspoon pepper

Sauté mushrooms, onion, and garlic in margarine until onion is golden. Place spinach on top of mushroom mixture and cover. Stir now and then. Cook until spinach is heated through (8-9 minutes); then stir in sour cream, salt, and pepper.

*GREEN BEAN SPECIAL

Exchanges per serving: 1 serving = 1/2 fat, 1 "A" vegetable.
Calories per serving: 50   Yield: 6 servings

1 teaspoon bacon chips	1 tomato, chopped
1 clove garlic, minced fine	2 1/2 cups green beans
1/4 cup onion, chopped fine	1 1/4 teaspoons salt
2 tablespoons green pepper,	1/8 teaspoon pepper
chopped fine	1/2 teaspoon oregano
1/3 cup water	

In skillet sauté bacon until lightly brown. Add garlic, onion, and pepper and sauté until onions are golden. Stir in tomato, green beans, salt, pepper, oregano, and water. Cover. Cook gently until beans are tender (about 15 minutes).

*GREEN BEANS DE LUXE

Exchanges per serving: 1 serving = 1 fat, 1 "A" vegetable.
Calories per serving: 45   Yield: 6 servings

4 cups green beans	2 tablespoons diet margarine
1/4 cup mint flakes, dried	1/16 teaspoon salt
Non-nutritive sweetener	1/16 teaspoon pepper
equivalent to 1 tablespoon	
sugar	

Heat beans and mint flakes with sweetener to boiling point. Drain. Stir in rest of ingredients.

*ASPARAGUS WITH HERBS

Exchanges per serving: 1 serving = 1 fat, 1 "A" vegetable.
Calories per serving: 45   Yield: 3 servings

1 1/4 cups asparagus
1 tablespoon diet margarine
1/2 teaspoon salt

1/4 cup water
2 tablespoons chives, chopped
1/16 teaspoon seasoned salt

1/16 teaspoon pepper

Separate asparagus. Place margarine, salt, water, and chives in skillet and cover tightly. Bring to boil. Add asparagus and cover. Gently boil until asparagus is tender. Sprinkle with seasoned salt and pepper.

*PEAS AND LETTUCE

Exchanges per serving: 1 serving = 1 fat, 1 "A" and 1 "B" vegetable.
Calories per serving: 75   Yield: 4 servings

1 1/4 cups frozen peas
1 cup lettuce, chopped
coarsely

4 tablespoons diet margarine
(or omit margarine and delete fat exchange)

Cook peas in boiling salted water until tender (5-6 minutes). Add lettuce and simmer until wilted and transparent. Drain. Toss with margarine or butter.

*BEETS WILLIAM-STYLE

Exchanges per serving: 1 serving = 1 "B" vegetable.
Calories per serving: 35   Yield: 4 servings

Non-nutritive sweetener
equivalent to 2 tablespoons
sugar
1/2 teaspoon salt

1/2 teaspoon pepper
3/4 teaspoon arrowroot powder
2 cups sliced beets

2 tablespoons lemon juice

Mix sweetener, salt, pepper, and arrowroot powder. Drain liquid from beets, saving 1/3 cup. Stir the 1/3 cup liquid with lemon juice and drained beets into sweetened mixture. Boil until sauce thickens and beets are heated. Stir constantly.

*TOMATOES WITH CHEESE TOPPING

Exchanges per serving: 1 serving = 1/4 meat, 1 "A" vegetable.
Calories per serving: 20   Yield: 4 servings

2 tomatoes, peeled and halved
1/2 teaspoon thyme
2 tablespoons American
cheese, grated fine

2 tablespoons seasoned dried
bread crumbs
1/2 teaspoon salt
1/8 teaspoon pepper

Preheat oven to 375°. Place tomatoes, cut side up, in baking pan and top each half with a mixture of thyme, cheese, bread crumbs, salt, and pepper. Bake until tomatoes are tender and cheese melts (about 20 minutes). Put baking pan under broiler for the last minute or so to brown tops.

*CELERY AND CARROTS (WITH HORSERADISH)

Exchanges per serving: 1 serving = 1/2 fat, 1 "A" and 1 "B" vegetable.
Calories per serving: 55
Yield: 6 servings

2 cups carrots, cut into 1/2" slices
2/3 cup celery, cut into 1/2" pieces
1 cup water
1 1/2 teaspoons prepared horseradish
1/2 teaspoon salt
2 tablespoons diet margarine

Scrape carrots before slicing; remove any strings from celery and slice. After slicing, place carrots and celery in tightly covered saucepan and boil in water with horseradish and salt until tender (about 20 minutes). Drain and add margarine.

*SWEET CARROTS

Exchanges per serving: 2/3 cup = 1 fat, 1 "B" vegetable.
Calories per serving: 80
Yield: 2 cups

1 tablespoon diet margarine
2 tablespoons water
1/2 teaspoon salt
1/8 teaspoon pepper
Non-nutritive sweetener equivalent to 1/2 teaspoon sugar
2 tablespoons parsley, snipped fine
2 cups carrots, scraped and sliced thin

Melt margarine; add rest of ingredients. Cover. Simmer gently about 10 minutes. Stir occasionally.

*GINGERED CARROTS

Exchanges per serving: 1 serving = 1/2 fat, 1 "B" vegetable.
Calories per serving: 55
Yield: 2 1/2 cups

2 cups carrots, julienne
1/2 cup water
1/2 teaspoon Mei Yen Seasoning
1/2 teaspoon ginger
Non-nutritive sweetener equivalent to 1/2 teaspoon sugar
2 tablespoons diet margarine

Cook carrots in water seasoned with Mei Yen powder; add ginger, sweetener, and when tender, margarine. Continue to cook 3-4 minutes. Stir gently.

*CARROTS WITH ORANGE

Exchanges per serving: 1/2 cup = 1/2 fat, 1 fruit, 1 "B" vegetable.
Calories per serving: 98   Yield: 6 servings

Water to cover carrots
3 teaspoons salt
3 cups carrots, scraped and
    sliced thin

Non-nutritive sweetener
    equivalent to 1 tablespoon
    sugar
2 tablespoons diet margarine
4 oranges, cut into sections

Place 2 teaspoons salt in water; gently boil carrots until tender; add remaining salt, sweetener, margarine, and oranges. Heat slowly and gently.

**DELIGHTFUL CARROTS

Exchanges per serving: 1 serving = 1 1/2 fat, 1 "B" vegetable.
Calories per serving: 103   Yield: 4 servings

6 carrots, peeled and cut into
    3" strips
4 tablespoons diet margarine
1 tablespoon lemon juice

1/8 teaspoon celery seed
1/2 teaspoon salt
2 tablespoons water

Preheat oven to 350°. Arrange carrots in small baking dish; melt margarine, then combine with remaining ingredients. Pour over carrots. Cover and bake about 3/4 hour (or until carrots are tender).

**CARROTS WITH CHEESE

Exchanges per serving: 1 cup = 1 meat, 1 "B" vegetable.
Calories per serving: 105   Yield: 2 cups

2 cups carrots, sliced
1/2 cup cheese, grated
1/8 teaspoon salt

1/8 teaspoon pepper
1/16 cup parsley flakes

Boil carrots gently about 5 minutes; turn off heat and drain thoroughly. Return to saucepan. Sprinkle with cheese, letting carrots stay on burner until cheese melts. Sprinkle with salt and pepper and top with parsley.

**PINEAPPLE SWEET POTATOES

Exchanges per serving: 1 serving = 1 bread, 1/2 fat, 1 fruit.
Calories per serving: 135   Yield: 8 servings

8 sweet potatoes
1 1/2 teaspoons salt
1/8 teaspoon pepper

2 cups artificially sweetened
    pineapple tidbits
2 tablespoons diet margarine

Boil potatoes until tender; cool slightly. Mash until smooth; stir in rest of ingredients, including syrup from pineapple tidbits. Return to stove and reheat.

**BAKED POTATOES, STUFFED

Exchanges per serving: 1 potato = 1 bread, 2 fat.
Calories per serving: 150   Yield: 8 servings

8 potatoes	1 1/2 teaspoons salt
1 tablespoon oil	1/8 teaspoon pepper
1 1/2 cups sour cream	2 tablespoons chives, snipped

Preheat oven to 450°. Prick skins of potatoes with fork, lightly oil your hands and rub the oil onto the potatoes. Place potatoes in oven and bake until done (about 35-40 minutes). Reduce heat to 325°. Remove potatoes from oven and cut a thin slice from each and hollow out, being sure to leave shell intact. Mash centers in electric mixer with sour cream, salt, pepper, and chives; refill shells, heaping high. Bake on aluminum foil until heated through and potato top is lightly browned (about 1/2 hour).

**ANNE'S STUFFED BAKED POTATOES WITH CHEESE

Exchanges per serving: 1 potato = 1 bread, 1 fat, 1 meat.
Calories per serving: 186   Yield: 8 servings

8 potatoes	1/16 teaspoon salt
5 tablespoons diet margarine	1/16 teaspoon pepper
1/2 cup skim milk	1 cup cheese, finely grated

Preheat oven to 400°. Bake potatoes in oven until done (approximately 1 hour); while hot, cut tops off and scoop insides into mixing bowl, keeping the 8 shells. Add margarine and skim milk and beat until smooth. Add rest of ingredients and continue beating until mixed thoroughly. Refill potato shells, place on baking dish for 20 minutes, then under broiler until delicately browned.

**MARGE'S STUFFED POTATOES

Exchanges per serving: 1 potato = 1 bread, 1 fat.
Calories per serving: 115   Yield: 6 servings

6 potatoes	3 1/2 tablespoons Parmesan cheese, grated
1 teaspoon salt	1/2 teaspoon pepper
1 tablespoon chives, chopped fine	1 tablespoon imitation sour cream
2 tablespoons bacon bits	1/16 teaspoon paprika
1/2 cup diet margarine	

Preheat oven to 400°. Grease, then bake potatoes until soft. Cut in half lengthwise. Spoon out centers while hot, saving skins, and put centers in mixing bowl. Add rest of ingredients except paprika to bowl and mix about 3 minutes at medium speed with electric mixer. Place mixture in potato skins. Sprinkle lightly with paprika and brown in oven about 4 minutes.

**POLLY'S CREAMED POTATOES

Exchanges per serving: 1 serving = 1 bread, 1 fat, 1/2 milk, 1 "A"
                       vegetable.
Calories per serving: 200   Yield: 8 servings

8 potatoes, pared and cubed	2 1/2 cups milk
1 onion, sliced thin	2 tablespoons diet margarine
1 cup celery, sliced thin	1/8 cup water
3/4 tablespoon chervil	1/2 tablespoon arrowroot
2 teaspoons salt	powder
1/8 teaspoon pepper	2 tablespoons dried parsley

Mix everything except the water, arrowroot and parsley in saucepan
and cook until potatoes are tender (20-25 minutes). Mix arrowroot and
water to make a thin paste and stir into first mixture. Cover and cook
until thick and smooth, stirring occasionally. Garnish with parsley.

**SUPER RICE

Exchanges per serving: 1 serving = 1 bread, 1 fat.
Calories per serving: 115   Yield: 8 servings

1 cup uncooked white rice	Non-nutritive sweetener
1/4 teaspoon lemon juice	equivalent to 1 tablespoon
1 cup + 2 tablespoons frozen	sugar
peas	1 onion, diced fine
	2 tablespoons salad oil
	1/2 teaspoon parsley flakes

Cook rice according to the directions on the package, but substitute
lemon juice for butter. Cook peas, add sweetener. In a skillet sauté
onion in oil until wilted and golden. Add the peas and onion to rice.
Garnish with parsley.

BREADS

*STUFFING
(For chicken, meat, or turkey)

Exchanges per serving: 1 cup = 1/2 bread, 1/2 fat.
Calories per serving: 57

Yield: 3 1/4 cups

1/2 cup celery, chopped fine
1/2 cup onion, chopped fine
1/2 cup mushrooms, chopped fine

1/4 cup diet margarine
1 cup herb-seasoned stuffing mix
1 cup boiling water

Sauté celery, onion, and mushrooms in margarine until onion is golden. Add stuffing mix to boiling water, then toss all together. Mix well.

*BERRY MUFFINS

Exchanges per serving: 1 muffin = 1 bread.
Calories per serving: 68

Yield: 12 muffins

2 cups biscuit mix
Non-nutritive sweetener equivalent to 1/4 cup + 2 tablespoons sugar
1 cup unflavored yogurt

1/4 cup (1 medium) egg
1 cup berries (blueberries, raspberries, etc.)
2 teaspoons lemon peel, grated

Preheat oven to 425°. Grease 12 muffin cups (2 1/2") and place in muffin pan. Combine mix and all but 2 tablespoons of sweetener in bowl; add yogurt. Add egg, beat with fork until well combined. Fold berries gently into batter with rubber spatula, then place about 1/4 cup batter into each cup. Combine lemon peel and remaining sweetener and mix well. Sprinkle over batter in each cup. Bake until golden brown (20-25 minutes). Serve hot.

*EASY RAISIN BREAD

Exchanges per serving: 1 serving = 1 bread.
Calories per serving: 68

Yield: 15 servings

1/2 cup quick-cooking oatmeal
1 teaspoon baking powder
2 cups biscuit mix
1/4 teaspoon salt
1/2 cup white raisins

1/4 cup (1 medium) egg, well beaten
1 1/4 cups skim milk
Non-nutritive sweetener equivalent to 4/5 cup sugar

Preheat oven to 350°. Combine dry ingredients, then mix rest of ingredients and add to dry ingredients. Blend well. Pour into 1 quart-round casserole, which has been well greased. Bake until done (about 1 hour). Cool ten minutes before turning out on rack.

*PANCAKES

Exchanges per serving: 1 pancake = 1 bread.
Calories per serving: 70

Yield: 10 4-inch pancakes

1 1/4 cups flour
2 1/2 teaspoons baking powder
Non-nutritive sweetener
equivalent to 2 tablespoons
sugar

3/4 teaspoon salt
1/4 cup (1 medium) egg
1 1/4 cups skim milk
2 tablespoons diet margarine,
melted

Mix and sift flour, baking powder, sweetener, and salt in medium bowl.
In another bowl beat egg, stir in skim milk and margarine; stir into
flour mixture until dry ingredients are wet. Heat pan until water
dropped on it "jumps" up and down. For each pancake put about 3
tablespoons of mixture on pan and cook over low heat until bubbles
appear on top and underside is nicely browned. Turn with a spatula and
brown other side.

*SHORTBREAD

Exchanges per serving: 1" x 3" piece = 1/4 bread, 1 fat, 1/3 fruit.
Calories per serving: 73

Yield: 36 servings

1/2 cup diet margarine
Non-nutritive sweetener
equivalent to 1 1/2 cups
brown sugar
1 cup plus 2 tablespoons flour,
sifted
1/2 cup (2 medium) eggs

1 teaspoon vanilla extract
1 teaspoon orange peel, grated
1/2 teaspoon salt
1 teaspoon baking powder
1 1/2 cups white raisins,
chopped
1 cup nuts, chopped fine

Preheat oven to 375°. Mix margarine, 1/2 of the sweetener, and 1 cup
of flour together to fine crumbs, then press firmly in the bottom of a 2"
x 9" x 13" pan. Bake 10 minutes. Meanwhile beat eggs until fluffy, beat
in remaining sweetener, vanilla, and orange peel. Add remaining flour,
salt, and baking powder. Mix well. Stir in raisins and nuts, then place
over crust which has been slightly cooled. Place entire mixture in oven
and bake another 30 minutes. Cool slightly, then cut.

*JOAN'S BISCUITS

Exchanges per serving: 1 biscuit = 1 bread, 1/2 fat.
Calories per serving: 90   Yield: 16 biscuits

2 cups flour	3 teaspoons baking powder
1 teaspoon salt	1/4 cup diet margarine
	3/4 cup skim milk

Preheat oven to 450°. Sift flour, salt, and baking powder. Cut in margarine until well mixed with first ingredients, then add milk. Knead several times; roll out on lightly floured board until about 1/2" thick. Cut with biscuit cutter or inverted glass, or drop by spoonsful. Place on heavy-duty aluminum foil or cookie sheet which has been well greased. Bake until browned (13-14 minutes).

*BLINTZES WITH CHEESE FILLING

Exchanges per serving: 1 serving = 1/2 bread, 1/2 fat, 1/2 meat.
Calories per serving: 95   Yield: 12 servings

1 cup flour	1 cup nonfat creamed cottage
1/2 teaspoon baking powder	cheese, sieved
1/2 teaspoon salt	Non-nutritive sweetener
1 cup (4 medium) eggs	equivalent to 2 tablespoons
1 cup skim milk	sugar
2 tablespoons diet margarine	1/4 teaspoon cinnamon

Sift flour, baking powder, and salt together. Beat 1/2 cup eggs, skim milk, and half the margarine and slowly add to flour mixture. Stir to form smooth batter, which will be thin. Grease a pan with remaining margarine, lightly, then pour 1/8 cup batter into skillet. (Tilt pan so batter completely covers bottom.) Cook until top of pancake is dry and bubbly, then turn onto brown paper (or paper towel). Make another 11 pancakes. Grease skillet when necessary. Mix sieved cottage cheese, sweetener, cinnamon, and remaining 1/2 cup of eggs. Turn brown side of each pancake up and place 1 tablespoon of filling in center. Fold over sides, then ends, to seal; set to one side. Refrigerate until ready to serve. About 10 minutes before serving, melt some margarine in large skillet and, with flap side down, lightly brown each blintze; turn and brown other side. Serve warm.

**MARY C'S MUFFINS

Exchanges per serving: 1 muffin = 1 bread, 1 fat.
Calories per serving: 115   Yield: 24 servings

1/2 cup diet margarine
Non-nutritive sweetener
   equivalent to 2/3 cup sugar
3/4 cup (3 medium) eggs

4 cups flour
6 teaspoons baking powder
2 teaspoons salt
1 1/2 cups milk

Preheat oven to 400°. Cream margarine and sweetener well. Beat eggs and add. Sift flour, baking powder and salt together and add alternately with milk to creamed mixture. Fill well-greased muffin pans 2/3 full. Bake 45 minutes. Serve hot.

**"SEEDED" STUFFING
(For chicken, meat, turkey)

Exchanges per serving: 1/2 cup = 1 bread, 1 fat.
Calories per serving: 115   Yield: 6 cups

1 onion, chopped fine
2 stalks celery, chopped fine
1/4 pound mushrooms, chopped fine
2 tablespoons diet margarine

1 8-ounce package stuffing mix
1/4 teaspoon each, celery, sesame, and poppy seeds
1 cup boiling water

Sauté onion, celery, and mushrooms in margarine until onion is golden. Add stuffing mix and seeds to boiling water, then mix all ingredients together.

**WAFFLES

Exchanges per serving: 1 waffle = 1 bread, 1 fat.
Calories per serving: 115   Yield: 10 4-inch waffles

1 1/2 cups flour
2 teaspoons baking powder
1/2 teaspoon salt
1/2 cup (2 medium) eggs
1 1/4 cups skim milk

Non-nutritive sweetener
   equivalent to 1/4 cup sugar
3 tablespoons diet margarine, melted

Heat waffle iron. Sift dry ingredients into bowl. In another bowl beat eggs, skim milk, sweetener, and margarine. Stir mixtures together until flour is wet and batter nearly smooth. Allow 4 tablespoons of batter for each 4" waffle.

** "SEEDED" BREAD

Exchanges per serving: 1 slice = 1 bread, 1 fat.
Calories per serving: 102   Yield: 1 slice

1 slice bread
1 teaspoon diet margarine
1/4 teaspoon celery seeds

1/2 teaspoon poppy seeds
1/4 teaspoon sesame seeds
1/16 teaspoon garlic salt

Spread bread with margarine. Sprinkle with combination of seeds, then
garlic salt. Put under broiler until edges of bread are brown and
margarine melted. Serve hot or cold.

**BARB'S POPOVERS

Exchanges per serving: 1 popover = 1 bread, 1/2 fat.
Calories per serving: 104   Yield: 16 popovers

1 cup (4 medium) eggs
2 cups skim milk
2 cups flour, sifted

1/2 teaspoon salt
2 tablespoons diet margarine,
  melted

Heat oven to 425°. Beat eggs, add milk while beating. Slowly add flour
and salt. Continue to beat to prevent lumps, then add melted margarine. Pour batter into cups which have been well greased. Bake 3/4
hour.

**SOUR CREAM MUFFINS

Exchanges per serving: 1 muffin = 1 bread, 3 fat.
Calories per serving: 195   Yield: 8 muffins

1/4 cup diet margarine
3/4 cup imitation sour cream
1 1/3 cups sifted all-purpose
  flour
Non-nutritive sweetener
  equivalent to 1/2 cup sugar

1/2 teaspoon baking soda
1/4 teaspoon salt
1/16 teaspoon nutmeg
1/4 cup (1 medium) egg, beat-
  en

Preheat oven to 450°. Cream margarine; add sour cream. Mix well. Sift
dry ingredients. Add alternately with egg to first mixture. Spoon into
greased muffin tins and bake for 15 minutes.

**CORNMEAL BERRY MUFFINS

Exchanges per serving: 1 muffin = 1 bread, 1 fat.
Calories per serving: 113   Yield: 15 muffins

1/3 cup diet margarine, melted
Non-nutritive sweetener equivalent to 1/3 cup sugar
1/4 cup water
1/2 cup (2 medium) eggs
1 1/4 cups cornmeal

3/4 cup flour
2 1/2 teaspoons baking powder
1/4 teaspoon salt
3/4 cup milk
2/3 cup berries (blueberries, blackberries, etc.)

Preheat oven to 400°. Beat together the margarine, sweetener, water, and eggs, then stir in cornmeal. Sift flour, baking powder, and salt. Stir 1/4 of this into first mixture with 1/4 of the milk. Repeat until used. Wash and drain berries and fold gently into batter. Place about 4 tablespoons in each muffin cup which has been well greased. Bake until brown and separated from edge of cups (about 20 minutes).

**DATE BREAD

Exchanges per serving: 1 slice = 1 bread, 1/2 fat, 1/2 fruit.
Calories per serving: 113   Yield: 24 servings

3 cups flour, sifted
1 1/2 teaspoons salt
1/2 teaspoon ground cloves
1/2 teaspoon nutmeg
4 1/2 teaspoons baking powder
1 teaspoon mace
1/2 teaspoon allspice
2 dozen dates, chopped well

1 cup skim milk
Non-nutritive sweetener equivalent to 1 1/2 cups sugar
1/2 cup (2 medium) eggs, well beaten
1/4 cup diet margarine, melted

Preheat oven to 350°. Sift first seven ingredients. Add dates; mix skim milk, sweetener, eggs, and margarine and add to first mixture. Place in 3" x 5" x 9" loaf pan which has been well greased. Bake 1 hour and 15 minutes.

**CORNBREAD

Exchanges per serving: 1 square = 1 bread, 1 fat.
Calories per serving: 113 				Yield: 9 servings

1 1/4 cups flour
3/4 cup yellow cornmeal
Non-nutritive sweetener equivalent to 2 tablespoons sugar
4 1/2 teaspoons baking powder

1 teaspoon salt
1/4 cup (one medium) egg
2/3 cup milk
1/3 cup diet margarine, melted

Preheat oven to 425°. Sift everything except eggs, milk, and margarine into small bowl. Beat eggs well, stir in milk and margarine. Pour into flour mixture all at once; stir until flour is just moistened (mixture will be lumpy). Put into pan which has been well greased. Spread evenly and bake until bread comes away from edges of pan (about 1/2 hour). Cut into equal squares.

**RAISIN BREAD

Exchanges per serving: 1 1/2" slice = 1 bread, 1 fat, 1/2 fruit, 1/2 meat.
Calories per serving: 168 				Yield: 16 servings

3 cups flour
3 1/2 teaspoons baking powder
Non-nutritive sweetener equivalent to 3/4 cup sugar
1 1/2 teaspoons salt
1/3 cup diet margarine

2 teaspoons orange peel, grated
1/2 cup (2 medium) eggs
1 cup skim milk
1 cup white raisins, chopped
1/2 cup nuts, chopped fine

Preheat oven to 350°. Sift dry ingredients; add margarine, orange peel, egg, and skim milk. Mix until blended, then stir in raisins and nuts. Place in 3" x 5" x 9" loaf pan which has been well greased. Bake 1 hour and 15 minutes or until loaf tests done. Remove from pan. Cool and store 12 hours before slicing.

**BARBARA'S BANANA BREAD

Exchanges per serving: 1 serving = 1 bread, 1 fat, 1/3 fruit.
Calories per serving: 130

Yield: 12 servings

1/4 teaspoon baking soda
1/2 teaspoon salt
1 3/4 cups flour
2 teaspoons baking powder
1/4 cup diet margarine, melted

1/4 cup (1 medium) egg, well
beaten
Non-nutritive sweetener
equivalent to 1 cup sugar
1 teaspoon almond extract
2 bananas, mashed well

Preheat oven to 350°. Sift dry ingredients together. Combine margarine, eggs, sweetener, and almond extract; add to first mixture, stirring
until flour is moistened. Fold in mashed bananas. Turn into loaf pan
which has been well greased. Bake until done (about 1 hour).

**BANANA BREAD

Exchanges per serving: 1 slice = 1 bread, 1 fat, 1/4 fruit.
Calories per serving: 135

Yield: 30 servings

3 1/4 cups flour
4 teaspoons baking powder
1 teaspoon salt
1/2 teaspoon baking soda
1/2 cup diet margarine, melted

1 cup (4 medium) eggs, well
beaten
Non-nutritive sweetener
equivalent to 4 cups sugar
2 teaspoons vanilla extract
4 bananas, mashed well

Preheat oven to 350°. Sift flour, baking powder, salt, and baking soda.
Mix margarine, eggs, sweetener, and vanilla. Add to flour mixture and
stir until flour is moistened, then fold in mashed bananas. Place in 3" x
4" x 8" loaf pan which has been well greased. Bake 1 hour and 10
minutes.

**LEMON MUFFINS

Exchanges per serving: 1 muffin = 1 bread, 1 fat.
Calories per serving: 120

Yield: 12 muffins

2 cups all-purpose flour, sifted
1/2 cup sugar
3 teaspoons baking powder
1/2 teaspoon salt

2/3 cup skim milk
1/3 cup lemon juice
1 teaspoon lemon rind, grated
1/3 cup salad oil

1/4 cup (1 medium) egg, slightly beaten

Preheat oven to 400°. Grease muffin tins. Sift flour, sugar, baking
powder, and salt into a large bowl. Combine milk, lemon juice, lemon
rind, oil, and egg and beat with a fork to mix well. Pour wet into dry
ingredients; stir quickly with fork (do not beat—batter will be lumpy).
Fill each muffin cup slightly more than half full. Bake 20-25 minutes or
until golden (or until cake tester comes out clean). Remove from oven,
loosen edge of muffins with spatula, and turn out.

**AUNT JEANNE'S COFFEE CAKE

Exchanges per serving: 1 serving = 1 1/2 bread, 1 fat.
Calories per serving: 155   Yield: 8 servings

2 cups flour	3 drops yellow food coloring
3 teaspoons baking powder	Non-nutritive sweetener
1/4 teaspoon salt	equivalent to 1/2 cup plus 4
1/3 cup diet margarine, softened	teaspoons sugar
	1/4 cup (1 medium) egg
3/4 cup skim milk	1/2 teaspoon cinnamon

1/4 cup bread crumbs, toasted

Preheat oven to 375°. Sift flour, baking powder, and salt into small bowl; with electric beater, cut in 3 tablespoons of margarine on lowest speed, then turn to medium speed for about 5 minutes until well blended and resembling small peas. Add 1/2 cup of skim milk mixed with coloring and all but 4 teaspoons of sweetener. Continue beating on medium speed for about one minute. Batter will be stiff. Add rest of skim milk and beat for a minute, then add unbeaten egg and beat one more minute. Pour into a greased 8" round cake pan. Mix remaining tablespoon of margarine, cinnamon, and toasted bread crumbs and sprinkle on top of dough. Bake until cake springs back when lightly touched (about 20 minutes).

**MARVELOUS MARMALADE STUFFING

Exchanges per serving: 1/2 cup = 1 bread, 2 fat.
Calories per serving: 160   Yield: 3 cups

1 cup cornbread stuffing	1/4 cup onions, chopped fine
1/2 cup diet margarine, melted	1/4 cup almonds, slivered and chopped
1/2 cup celery, chopped fine	1/2 cup dietetic marmalade

Mix all ingredients. Toss lightly but thoroughly. Use to lightly stuff a 4-5 pound chicken.

**PAULA'S POPOVERS

Exchanges per serving: 1 popover = 1 bread, 1 fat.
Calories per serving: 125   Yield: 8 popovers

2 cups flour	1 cup (4 medium) eggs
1 teaspoon salt	2 cups milk

6 tablespoons diet margarine

Preheat oven to 350°. Sift flour and salt. Beat eggs slightly, add milk and margarine and beat until blended. Gradually add dry ingredients. Grease ramekin cups well and fill about 3/4 full. Bake 1 hour and 10 minutes, then remove from oven. Slit each side quickly to release steam. Return to oven until brown and crisp and tops are firm. Lift out of ramekins; serve hot.

**DATE AND NUT BREAD

Exchanges per serving: 1/4" slice = 1 bread, 1 fat, 1/2 fruit.
Calories per serving: 133   Yield: 2 loaves

4 cups dates, pitted
2 cups nuts, coarsely chopped
2 cups boiling water
2 3/4 cups flour
1 1/2 teaspoons baking soda
1 teaspoon salt

1/2 cup diet margarine, softened
Non-nutritive sweetener equivalent to 1 1/4 cups brown sugar, firmly packed
1/2 cup (2 medium) eggs
1 teaspoon vanilla extract

Preheat oven to 350°. Cut dates into small pieces with scissors. Add nuts and boiling water. Allow to cool to room temperature (about 3/4 hour). Sift flour with the baking soda and salt. On high speed of mixer beat margarine with sweetener, eggs, and vanilla until smooth; then add date mixture and mix well. Add flour mixture. Beat with wooden spoon until well combined. Place in 2 well-greased loaf pans. Bake 70 minutes, or until tester inserted in center of bread comes out clean. Cool 10 minutes in pan, then on wire rack until room temperature.

**BUTTERMILK BISCUITS WITH SEEDS

Exchanges per serving: 1 biscuit = 1 fat, 1 bread.
Calories per serving: 115   Yield: 24 servings

4 cups flour
4 teaspoons baking powder
1/2 teaspoon baking soda
2 teaspoons salt

2 tablespoons seeds (sesame, caraway, etc.)
1 1/2 cups skim buttermilk
2/3 cup safflower oil

Preheat oven to 350°. Sift the flour, baking powder, baking soda, and salt into bowl, then add seeds. Add buttermilk to oil but do not stir together; pour all at once over dry ingredients. Mix with fork to make soft dough. Turn dough onto floured board and knead lightly until smooth; flatten slightly, then cover with sheet of waxed paper; roll until about 1/4" thick, then remove paper. Cut a 6" x 8" rectangle into 2" squares. Bake until brown.

***PRUNE BREAD

Exchanges per serving: 1 slice = 2 bread, 1 fat, 1 fruit, 1/2 meat.
Calories per serving: 236   Yield: 12 slices

2 cups dried prunes
1 1/2 cups boiling water
3 cups flour
Non-nutritive sweetener
equivalent to 1 1/2 cups
sugar

1 teaspoon salt
2 teaspoons baking soda
1/2 cup (2 medium) eggs
4 tablespoons salad oil

Preheat oven to 325°. Put prunes to soak in cold water for two hours.
Drain and then pit and chop prunes. Add boiling water and let stand 5
minutes. Sift flour, sweetener, salt, and baking soda. Add prune
mixture. Beat and add eggs, then add salad oil. Pour into 2 greased loaf
pans 2 1/2" x 4 1/2" x 8 1/2" and bake for 1 hour. Remove from pans
and cool on wire rack.

***COFFEE CAKE, CHOCOLATE STYLE

Exchanges per serving: 1 half-inch slice = 3 bread, 1/4 fat, 1/4 meat.
Calories per serving: 245   Yield: 12 servings

2/3 cup diet margarine
Non-nutritive sweetener
equivalent to 1 cup sugar
3/4 cup (3 medium) eggs
1 teaspoon orange peel, grated
1 cup artificial sour cream
1 teaspoon vanilla extract
1/4 teaspoon salt
1/2 teaspoon baking soda

2 cups + 2 tablespoons flour
1 1/2 teaspoons baking powder
1 ounce unsweetened chocolate
Non-nutritive sweetener
equivalent to 1/2 cup brown
sugar
1 teaspoon cinnamon

1 tablespoon diet margarine

Preheat oven to 350°. Cream margarine and sweetener until light and
fluffy; add eggs one at a time. Beat until smooth. Mix orange peel, sour
cream, and vanilla. Stir salt, baking soda, baking powder, and two cups
of flour together, then blend with creamed mixture thoroughly. Place in
a well-greased, 10" tube pan. Melt chocolate in aluminum foil and swirl
over batter with spoon to form ripples through batter. Mix sugar
substitute, cinnamon, and softened margarine with remaining 2 tablespoons of flour and sprinkle over batter. Bake until straw inserted in
center comes out clean (50-60 minutes).

FRUITS AND FRUIT DESSERTS

*LUCY'S LUSCIOUS APRICOT SOUFFLE DESSERT

Exchanges per serving: 1 serving = 1/2 fruit.
Calories per serving: 20   Yield: 8 servings

1 cup dried apricots
Non-nutritive sweetener
  equivalent to 1 1/4 cups
  sugar
Water to cover

2 cups (12 medium) egg whites
1/16 teaspoon salt
1 cup nondairy whipping
  cream

Preheat oven to 300°. Combine apricots and sweetener equivalent to
3/4 cup sugar in a saucepan; add sufficient water to cover. Cook slowly
until sweetener dissolves, stirring occasionally, then cover pan and cook
over low heat until apricots are tender and plump. Drain. Retain syrup;
puree apricots. Beat egg whites, which should be at room temperature,
with salt until egg whites are stiff; add rest of sweetener. Fold in pureed
apricots, mixing thoroughly. Turn into buttered tube pan. Bake 3/4
hour. The soufflé will raise and become golden brown. Top with nondairy whip to which 2 tablespoons of apricot syrup have been added
after whipping.

*BAKED FRESH PEACHES

Exchanges per serving: 1 peach = 1 fruit.
Calories per serving: 40   Yield: 4 servings

4 peaches
1 teaspoon diet margarine

Non-nutritive sweetener
  equivalent to 1/2 cup sugar
1 tablespoon lemon juice

Preheat oven to 350°. Cut about an inch of skin from each end of peach
and set in a baking dish that has been well greased with the margarine.
Sprinkle with sweetener and lemon juice. Bake about 20 minutes; serve
cold or hot, with milk or cream if desired.

*BANANA FREEZE

Exchanges per serving: 1 cup = 1 fruit.
Calories per serving: 40   Yield: 6 cups

3 bananas, crushed
1 cup unsweetened orange
  juice

Non-nutritive sweetener
  equivalent to 2 tablespoons
  sugar
1 teaspoon lemon juice
1/4 cup water

Combine all ingredients, mixing well. Using paper cups, divide mixture
evenly into 6 and freeze until firm. Let stand at room temperature a few
minutes (5-6) and then peel paper cup as it is being eaten.

*FRUIT COCKTAIL CAKE DESSERT

Exchanges per serving: 1 = 1/2 bread, 1/2 fruit, 1/2 skim milk.
Calories per serving: 95   Yield: 10 servings

Non-nutritive sweetener
  equivalent to 1/2 cup sugar
1 tablespoon unflavored gelatin
1/4 teaspoon salt
1/2 cup water
4 cups dietetic fruit cocktail
1 tablespoon lemon juice

4-5 drops almond extract
1/4 cup (2 small) egg whites
1 cup nonfat dry milk,
  whipped
8 ladyfingers, split (these can
  be made from dietetic
  sponge cake)

Combine sweetener, gelatin, and salt. Add 1/2 cup water and cook,
stirring over medium heat until gelatin dissolves. Chill until partially
set; drain fruit cocktail, add lemon juice and almond extract. Put
gelatin mixture, egg whites, and half the fruit cocktail in a large mixing
bowl. Start mixer on low speed, then turn to high and beat 10 minutes,
until fluffy. Chill until partially set. Fold in remaining fruit cocktail and
whipped milk. Line sides of spring pan with ladyfingers. Pour filling in
carefully. Chill overnight. Remove sides of pan.

*APPLESAUCE, UNCOOKED

Exchanges per serving: 1 cup = 2 fruit.
Calories per serving: 80   Yield: 4 cups

2 cups apples, washed, cored,
  and cubed, but not peeled
2 cups cold water
3 tablespoons lemon juice
1/16 teaspoon cloves
1/16 teaspoon ginger

1/4 teaspoon nutmeg
Non-nutritive sweetener
  equivalent to 3 teaspoons
  sugar
2 drops red vegetable food
  coloring (optional)

Place apples in bowl which contains mixture of water and lemon juice.
Remove 1/2 cup of the juice from bowl and to it add sweetener and
spices and half the apple cubes. Blend, then add the additional cubes
gradually until all smoothly blended. Add coloring.

*SPICED FRUIT

Exchanges per serving: 1 cup = 2 fruit.
Calories per serving: 80   Yield: 5 cups

1 cup dietetic pineapple juice
1/4 teaspoon cinnamon

2 cups dietetic pear halves
2 cups dietetic peach halves

Heat pineapple juice and cinnamon to boil; chill fruit, from which syrup
has been drained, and place in a bowl. Pour pineapple juice over fruit,
then serve at once.

*DIETETIC SPICED PEACHES

Exchanges per serving: 1 serving = 1 fruit.
Calories per serving: 40   Yield: 2 servings

4 dietetic peach halves   1 cup liquid from peaches
16 whole cloves

Preheat oven to 375°. Place peaches in small pan, pitted side up. Stick 4 cloves in each half, then pour liquid over fruit. Bake 20 minutes. Serve hot.

*SUMMER FRUIT MIX

Exchanges per serving: 3/4 cup = 1 1/2 fruit.
Calories per serving: 60   Yield: 5 cups

2 cups strawberries   1 cup blueberries
1 cup grapes   Non-nutritive sweetener
1 cup melon balls   equivalent to 1/4 cup sugar

Wash and clean fruit, then combine with sweetener. Chill. This goes well topped with Custard Sauce for Shortcakes.

*BAKED APPLES

Exchanges per serving: 1 apple = 1 fruit.
Calories per serving: 40   Yield: 2 servings

2 medium apples   1/16 teaspoon allspice
2 teaspoons lemon juice   2 tablespoons dietetic maple
1/16 teaspoon nutmeg   topping for each apple
1/16 teaspoon cinnamon

Preheat oven to 350°. Core apples and peel about 1/2 of each apple; sprinkle lemon juice over cut surfaces. Dust apple with mixture of nutmeg, cinnamon, and allspice. Fill cavity with dietetic maple topping; bake covered about 25 minutes. Remove cover and continue baking until apples are tender.

*TASTY APPLESAUCE

Exchanges per serving: 1 serving = 1/4 fruit, 1/2 meat.
Calories per serving: 45   Yield: 4 servings

4 teaspoons cinnamon   1/2 cup unsweetened ap-
1 teaspoon salt   plesauce
1 teaspoon vanilla   1/3 cup (2 medium) egg
Non-nutritive sweetener   whites
  equivalent to 1/4 cup sugar   1/16 teaspoon allspice

Stir first five ingredients together. Place in refrigerator until chilled. Before serving beat whites to form stiff peaks. Fold applesauce mix into whites and sprinkle with allspice.

*FRUIT WHIP

Exchanges per serving: 1 serving = 1/2 skim milk.
Calories per serving: 40   Yield: 6 servings

1 1/2 tablespoons unflavored gelatin	Non-nutritive sweetener equivalent to 1/4 cup sugar
3 cups skim milk	2 teaspoons any fruit extract

Sprinkle gelatin over skim milk in saucepan and cook over low heat until gelatin dissolves. Add sweetener and fruit extract. Chill in refrigerator until mixture is consistency of egg white. Remove from refrigerator and beat at highest speed of mixer until mixture is doubled in volume (this will be very fluffy). Place in a mold and refrigerate until set. May be garnished with slice of favorite fruit, if desired.

*OLGA'S FRUIT FESTIVAL
(Not for diabetics without consent of doctor.)

Exchanges per serving: 1 serving = 1/2 fat, 2 fruit.
Calories per serving: 100 + liqueur   Yield: 8 servings

2 cups strawberries, culled and washed	1/4 cup orange curaçao
3 cups fresh peaches, peeled and sliced	1/2 cup low-calorie topping whip (or artificial whipping cream)
2 cups seedless green grapes	
Non-nutritive sweetener equivalent to 2/3 cup sugar	1 ounce unsweetened chocolate, well grated

Sprinkle strawberries over peaches, then add grapes, sweetener, and curaçao. Refrigerate overnight. Prior to serving heat broiler; place fruit in heatproof dessert dishes and top with topping whip or artificial whipping cream. Sprinkle top with grated chocolate and place under broiler about 1/2 minute, or just until chocolate melts. Serve at once.

**WINE SAUCE WITH FRUIT
(Not for diabetics without consent of doctor.)

Exchanges per serving: 1 serving = 1 fat, 2 1/2 fruit.
Calories per serving: 165 + alcohol   Yield: 4 servings

4 cups apples, peeled and sliced (or substitute bananas, peaches, pears, etc.)	1/2 tablespoon arrowroot powder
2 tablespoons diet margarine	Non-nutritive sweetener equivalent to 1 cup sugar
1 cup red wine	1/16 teaspoon allspice

Brown apples in margarine. Add wine to arrowroot powder a little at a time to make a smooth paste. Add sweetener and cook over medium heat. Stir constantly until clear and thick, then add allspice. Pour over fruit slices and simmer a few minutes. Serve immediately.

***HAWAIIAN FRUIT FRITTERS

Exchanges per serving: 1 fritter = 1/4 bread, 4 fat, 1/2 fruit, 1/4 meat.
Calories per serving: 235

Yield: 7 servings

1/2 cup ((2 medium) eggs
1/2 cup skim milk
1/2 teaspoon seasoned salt
2 cups fresh pineapple (or papaya or banana)

2 cups cornflakes, finely crushed
1 1/2 cups safflower oil

Beat eggs, skim milk, and salt together; cut fruit into inch-long pieces and dip in egg mixture. Roll in cornflakes. Deep fry in oil until golden brown. Serve with Hot Soy Sauce Dip.

***LEMON PUDDING

Exchanges per serving: 1 cup = 3 fat, 2 meat.
Calories per serving: 281

Yield: 4 servings

Non-nutritive sweetener equivalent to 1 1/2 cups sugar
1/2 cup diet margarine

2 tablespoons lemon peel
2 cups (8-9 medium) eggs
1 cup lemon juice

Combine all ingredients in top of double boiler. Cook over boiling water until thick; stir occasionally. Cover and store in refrigerator until cool.

****POLLY'S PEAR DISH

Exchanges per serving: 1 serving = 1 bread, 1 fat, 1 1/2 fruit.
Calories per serving: 310

Yield: 8 servings

1/2 cup water
Non-nutritive sweetener equivalent to 1 cup sugar
1 tablespoon fresh lemon juice
8 fresh pears, pared, cored, and sliced thin

1 pie shell, unbaked
1 cup low-calorie apricot preserves
1/16 teaspoon nutmeg
1/16 teaspoon allspice

Preheat oven to 425°. Combine water, sweetener, and lemon juice in saucepan, then add pear slices a few at a time; cook gently until tender (about 5-6 minutes). Cool a little, then drain and save 1/4 cup liquid. Place pear slices in circle in unbaked pie shell which has been rolled out to fit a 12" pan. Bake until golden brown, then cool. Combine apricot preserves and reserved liquid in a saucepan, heat until bubbly, then force through sieve. Spoon this over pear slices to glaze, and sprinkle with nutmeg and allspice. Chill and serve.

PUDDINGS AND SPECIAL DESSERTS

*MOCHA SURPRISE

Exchanges per serving: 1 cup = None.
Calories per serving: 0

Yield: 3 cups

2 envelopes unflavored gelatin
1/2 cup cold water
3 cups very strong coffee
Non-nutritive sweetener
  equivalent to 1/3 cup sugar

1/2 teaspoon vanilla
1/16 teaspoon salt
3 tablespoons nonfat whipping
  cream

Soften the gelatin in the water in a medium-size pan. Heat. Stir constantly until dissolved, then stir in coffee, sweetener, vanilla, and salt. Pour into a 2" x 8" x 8" pan and chill 2 hours. Put gelatin through potato ricer (or sieve) and place in 3 dessert dishes. Decorate each with 1 tablespoon nonfat whipping cream.

*CHOCOLATE BISQUE CAPRI

Exchanges per serving: 1 = 1/2 fat, trace milk.
Calories per serving: 23 + ice cream

Yield: 16 servings

1/2 cup toasted almonds,
  chopped
1/3 cup toasted coconut,
  chopped

1/2 teaspoon almond extract
1 quart low-calorie chocolate
  ice cream

Combine almonds and coconut, but reserve 2 tablespoons for topping. Fold nuts and almond extract quickly into ice cream, which should be rather soft. Place in small paper dessert cups and sprinkle with topping. Keep in freezer until ready to serve.

*PEAR PUDDING DORIS

Exchanges per serving: 1 serving = 1/4 milk, 1/4 fruit.
Calories per serving: 50

Yield: 6 servings

6 tablespoons nonfat dry milk
1 cup water, ice cold
1 envelope unflavored gelatin
1 5-ounce jar low-calorie
  chocolate topping

1/3 cup (2 medium) egg
  whites
1 jar unsweetened pear halves

Dissolve dry milk in 3/4 cup water; on rest of water sprinkle gelatin to soften. Mix the milk with the gelatin. Stir over low heat until gelatin dissolves, then add chocolate topping. Cool until mixture thickens enough to mound on a spoon. Beat egg whites stiff. Fold in. Drain pears well and line dessert dishes. Add chocolate mixture and chill until firm.

*APRICOT OR PRUNE FRUIT SNOW

Exchanges per serving: 1 = 1/3 fat, 1 fruit.
Calories per serving: 63   Yield: 6 servings

1 envelope lemon-flavored low-calorie gelatin
1 cup boiling water
1 cup low-calorie juice (apple or apricot nectar)

1/8 cup (1 medium) egg white
6 pieces of unsweetened fruit (apricots or prunes)
3 teaspoons almonds, slivered

Dissolve gelatin in boiling water. Add juice, cool. Chill until syrupy. Add white of egg and beat until frothy. Fill dessert glass with snow, chill until firm; decorate each with apricot or prune; sprinkle 1/2 teaspoon slivered almonds over fruit.

*FRUIT CAKE PUDDING

Exchanges per serving: 1 = 1/3 bread, 1/2 meat, 1/4 skim milk.
Calories per serving: 85   Yield: 6 servings

3/4 cup (3 medium) eggs, separated
1 tablespoon fresh citrus fruit peel, grated
1/4 cup fresh citrus fruit juice

1 1/2 cups skim milk
Non-nutritive sweetener equivalent to 6 tablespoons sugar
1/4 cup flour, sifted
1/16 teaspoon salt

Preheat oven to 325°. Beat whites until stiff peaks form, then set aside. Add peel and juice of fruit to yolk, beating at medium speed until well blended. Add skim milk. Beat about 1 minute at low speed, then add rest of dry ingredients and beat again at low speed until smooth. Fold into egg whites. Place in custard cups; place cups in baking pan filled with about 1" water. Bake until lightly browned on top (about 3/4 hour). Serve hot or cold.

*FRUIT MOUNTAIN

Exchanges per serving: 1 = 1 fruit, 1/4 milk.
Calories per serving: 100   Yield: 6 servings

1 envelope low-calorie vanilla pudding and pie-filling mix
1 teaspoon almond extract

1 jar low-calorie cherry or apple pie filling
Cinnamon

Prepare pudding according to directions on the package but using nonfat milk. Add almond extract. Divide into dessert glasses. Cool. Top with pie filling and garnish with cinnamon.

*FRUIT SOUFFLE

Exchanges per serving: 1 = 1 1/2 fruit.
Calories per serving: 60   Yield: 6 servings

1 envelope unflavored gelatin
1 cup cold water
1 teaspoon lemon rind, grated
fine

2 cups unsweetened fruit (apples, pears, pineapple)

Sprinkle gelatin on 1/2 cup water; soften a few minutes. Stir over low heat about 3 minutes until gelatin is dissolved. Add rest of water, rind, and fruit. Chill until thick enough to mound on spoon. Beat until very light, then pour into a souffle dish and chill until firm.

*LOW-CALORIE COFFEE CREAM MOUSSE

Exchanges per serving: 1 serving = 1/4 meat.
Calories per serving: 100   Yield: 12 servings

2 envelopes unflavored gelatin
2 cups cold coffee, double strength
3/4 cup (3 medium) eggs, separated
Non-nutritive sweetener equivalent to 3/4 cup sugar

1 ounce semisweet chocolate chips
3 tablespoons rum or brandy flavoring
2 cups nondairy whipping cream

Sprinkle gelatin over 1 cup coffee in small bowl and let soften about 5 minutes. Using a rotary beater, beat egg yolks with sweetener equivalent to 1/2 cup sugar until light, using the top of a double boiler in which to beat them. Once light, beat in rest of coffee, chocolate chips, and softened gelatin. Stir constantly over simmering water until chocolate is melted and coats a metal spoon (about 10 minutes). Remove from heat. Stir in flavoring. Set top of double boiler in ice and cool, stirring often, until mixture becomes as thick as unbeaten egg white. Beat 1 cup of nondairy cream until stiff, place in refrigerator until needed. When gelatin is nearly thick, beat the egg whites until soft peaks form when beaters are raised; gradually beat in rest of sweetener, until whites are stiff and glossy. Fold gelatin mixture into whipped cream; fold in whites gently, until well blended. Place in large mold which has been rinsed well with cold water. Place in refrigerator until firm, 5-6 hours. Beat 1 cup cream stiff and place on top of mold. To unmold: run knife around edge of mold; invert over serving platter. Place hot, damp cloth over mold and shake gently to release. Lift off mold.

CAKES

*DELIGHTFUL CHEESECAKE

Exchanges per serving: 1 = 1/8 bread, 1/4 fruit, 1/2 meat.
Calories per serving: 55   Yield: 9 servings

4 tablespoons graham-cracker crumbs
2 envelopes unflavored gelatin
1/2 cup water
1 cup low-calorie pineapple tidbits
Juice from pineapple tidbits plus water to make 3/4 cup
1 1/2 cups nonfat cottage cheese
3/4 cup (3 medium) eggs, separated
1/4 cup skim milk
2 tablespoons unsweetened lemon juice
Non-nutritive sweetener equivalent to 1/2 cup sugar
1 teaspoon vanilla extract
1/4 teaspoon salt

Sprinkle 3 tablespoons of the graham-cracker crumbs on bottom of 9" pan. Set aside. Soften gelatin in 1/2 cup water. Bring the 3/4 cup juice to boil and stir in gelatin. Beat cottage cheese until nearly smooth, at highest speed on mixer (about 3-4 minutes). Add egg yolks, skim milk, lemon juice, sweetener, vanilla extract, and salt. Beat well. Blend in gelatin at low speed. Chill. Stir occasionally until mixture is thick, but not set (about 1 hour). Beat whites at highest speed until soft peaks form, then fold in gelatin mixture by hand. Spoon over crumbs in pan and sprinkle remaining tablespoon of crumbs over filling. Add pineapple tidbits on top and chill overnight in refrigerator.

*ORANGE CUPCAKES

Exchanges per serving: 1 cupcake = 1/2 bread, 1/2 fat.
Calories per serving: 58   Yield: 30 cupcakes

1/2 cup diet margarine
Non-nutritive sweetener equivalent to 1 cup sugar
1/2 cup (2 medium) eggs, beaten
2/3 cup orange juice, strained
1/4 teaspoon salt
2 cups flour
2 teaspoons baking powder

Preheat oven to 325°. Cream margarine and sweetener. Add other ingredients and beat one minute or longer in mixer at high speed. Pour into baking cups and set in muffin tins. Bake until brown. Cool and frost, if desired.

*MARY'S SPONGE CAKE

Exchanges per serving: 1 1/2" slice = 1/2 bread, 1/2 meat.
Calories per serving: 75   Yield: 12 servings

1 cup flour
1/4 cup nonfat dry milk
1 teaspoon baking powder
1/4 teaspoon salt
3/4 cup (3 medium) eggs

Non-nutritive sweetener equivalent to 8 teaspoons sugar
2 tablespoons fresh orange juice
1 teaspoon orange rind, grated
1/2 teaspoon cream of tartar

Preheat oven to 325°. Sift flour, dry milk, baking powder and salt together three times; beat 2 whole eggs and 3 yolks at top speed of mixer until quite thick and lemon-colored (this takes about 10 minutes). Reduce speed, add sweetener gradually, and orange juice; increase speed and beat until very light and fluffy (about 5-6 minutes). Add rind and beat a little more. Beat remaining egg white slightly, add cream of tartar and continue beating until whites hold a stiff peak. Let stand while completing next step. Very carefully fold sifted dry ingredients, a small amount at a time, into egg-sweetener mixture, using rubber spatula or wire whip. Then fold in egg-white mixture very carefully. Pour at once into 9" tube pan. (If pan has removable bottom, no need to do anything to pan as a knife will help loosen cake from bottom. Otherwise line just the bottom of pan with piece of thin waxed paper; moisten well with water to make it flat.) Bake about 35 minutes. Cake is done when it springs back when touched with finger. Cool in pan upside down and remove carefully.

*POLLY'S DIETETIC JELLY ROLL

Exchanges per serving: 1 = 1/2 bread, 1/2 meat.
Calories per serving: 75   Yield: 12 servings

3/4 cup (3 medium) eggs, separated
Non-nutritive sweetener equivalent to 1/3 cup sugar
2 teaspoons orange juice
4 teaspoons liquid from any dietetic fruit
1/2 teaspoon lemon extract

1/2 teaspoon lemon extract
1 cup flour
1/3 cup nonfat dry milk solids
1 teaspoon baking powder
1/4 teaspoon salt
1/2 teaspoon cream of tartar
1/2 cup dietetic jelly

Preheat oven to 325°. Mix eggs, sweetener, orange juice, liquid from fruit, and lemon extract. Beat about 10 minutes with electric beater until very light and fluffy. Sift flour, milk solids, baking powder, and salt together three times; very carefully fold sifted dry ingredients into whipped mixture. Beat remaining egg whites and cream of tartar together until mixture stands in soft peaks. Fold into cake mixture. Pour into jelly-roll pan (about 10" x 15") which has been lined with lightly greased wax paper. Bake about 20 minutes; cake will spring back when touched with finger. Remove from oven and run knife around edge. Turn out onto towel, remove paper carefully and roll up immediately. Let stand one minute, unroll to cool. Fill with jelly and reroll. Slice to serve. *NOTE:* Jelly roll must be kept in refrigerator. Any dietetic pudding mix may be used for filling. When pudding is set, beat and put in roll.

*BANANA RAISIN CAKE

Exchanges per serving: 1 inch and a half cube = 1/2 bread, 1/2 fat, 1/4 fruit.

Calories per serving: 80   Yield: 36 servings

2 cups flour
1 1/2 teaspoons baking powder
Non-nutritive sweetener
equivalent to 1 1/2 cups
sugar
1 teaspoon baking soda
1 teaspoon salt

1/2 cup diet margarine
1 cup (about 3) mashed bananas
1/4 cup skim milk
1 teaspoon lemon peel, grated
1 teaspoon vanilla extract
1/2 cup (2 medium) eggs
1 cup white raisins, chopped

1/2 cup nuts, chopped fine

Preheat oven to 350°. Sift flour, baking powder, sweetener, baking soda and salt. Add margarine, bananas, skim milk, lemon peel, and vanilla. Beat 3 minutes on electric mixer at medium speed, scrape bowl constantly. Add eggs, beat 2 minutes more, continuing to scrape bowl frequently. Stir in raisins and nuts. Place batter in a 2" x 9" x 12" pan which has been well greased and lightly floured. Bake until cake tests done. Turn out on rack to cool after 5 minutes.

*SPICE AND MAPLE CAKE

Exchanges per serving: 1 1/2" slice = 1/2 bread, 1/2 meat.
Calories per serving: 85
                                              Yield: 10 servings

1 cup flour
1/4 cup nonfat dry milk solids
1 teaspoon baking powder
1 teaspoon cinnamon
1 teaspoon nutmeg
1/4 teaspoon salt

1/2 cup (2 medium) eggs, separated
1/4 cup (3 medium) egg yolks
1/2 cup maple-flavored topping
1/2 teaspoon cream of tartar

Preheat oven to 325°. Sift dry ingredients together three times. Mix eggs and egg yolks with the maple topping. Beat at top speed of mixer until light and fluffy (about 10 minutes). Beat remaining whites slightly; add cream of tartar and continue to beat until whites hold stiff peak. Fold sifted dry ingredients carefully, a small amount at a time, into egg and maple topping mixture. Fold in egg whites; pour into 9" tube cake pan at once. Bake about 35 minutes, or until cake springs back when lightly touched. Invert pan at once and let hang until cool.

*AUNT JEANNE'S SPONGE CAKE

Exchanges per serving: 1/2" thick slice = 1/2 bread, 1/2 meat.
Calories per serving: 70   Yield: 20 servings

1 cup skim milk
1 3/4 cups flour
2 teaspoons baking powder
1/2 teaspoon salt

1 1/2 cups (6 medium) eggs
Non-nutritive sweetener
   equivalent to 2 cups sugar
2 teaspoons vanilla

Preheat oven to 350°. Heat skim milk in a small saucepan just until bubbles form around edge of pan. Remove from heat and put aside until lukewarm. Sift flour, baking powder, and salt. Beat eggs until thick and lemon-colored; gradually add sweetener, beating until mixture is well blended and smooth (4-5 minutes). Blend in flour mixture at low speed of mixer until smooth, then add lukewarm milk and vanilla. Continue beating until well mixed. Place batter in an ungreased 10" tube pan. Bake 50 minutes, or until tester inserted in center of cake comes out clean. Turn cake — and cake pan — upside down and place tube over the neck of a bottle. This allows air to circulate around top (upside down) of cake, cooling it. Serve with imitation strawberry ice cream.

*VANILLA SPONGE ROLL

Exchanges per serving: 1 serving = 1/3 bread, 2/3 meat.
Calories per serving: 66   Yield: 6 servings

1 cup (about 4 medium) eggs,
   separated
Non-nutritive sweetener
   equivalent to 4 tablespoons
   sugar

1 teaspoon baking powder
5 tablespoons potato flour
1 teaspoon vanilla

Preheat oven to 325°. Add sweetener to stiffly beaten egg whites. Fold in the yolks and the rest of the ingredients. Bake in oblong pan 10" x 15" lined with paper greased on both sides; fill and bake 40 minutes. Spread cake with dietetic jelly, roll, and dust with granulated sugar substitute.

*CHOCOLATE CAKE

Exchanges per serving: 1 = 3/4 bread, 3/4 fat.
Calories per serving: 70   Yield: 8 servings

3/4 cup flour, sifted
1/4 teaspoon salt
1 teaspoon baking powder
1/4 teaspoon baking soda
3 tablespoons unsweetened
   cocoa
1/4 cup cold coffee

1/4 cup (1 medium) egg
Non-nutritive sweetener
   equivalent to 1/2 cup sugar
1/4 cup water
1 tablespoon salad oil
1 teaspoon vanilla extract

Preheat oven to 350°. Line an 8" round layer cake pan with paper; grease with butter. Sift first four ingredients together; blend in cocoa and coffee. Beat egg, sweetener, water, oil, and vanilla. Stir into dry ingredients. Mix until smooth. Pour batter into pan, cover with foil, and place in shallow pan of water. Bake about 1/2 hour. Remove from pan and cool on cake rack. Cut crosswise, fill, and frost with desired frosting.

*FRUIT SPONGE CAKE

Exchanges per serving: 1 serving = 1 bread, 1/2 meat.
Calories per serving: 100   Yield: 12 servings

1 tablespoon fresh orange rind, grated
1/2 cup fresh orange juice
1 cup (4 medium) eggs, separated
Non-nutritive sweetener equivalent to 1/2 cup sugar
2 tablespoons fresh lemon juice
1/2 teaspoon vanilla extract
1 1/2 cups flour
1/4 teaspoon salt
3/4 teaspoon cream of tartar

Preheat oven to 325°. Combine rind and juice. Beat egg yolks until thick and lemon-colored using highest speed of mixer. To juice and rind of orange, add sweetener, lemon juice, and vanilla extract. Sift flour and salt together and beat into egg yolks, alternating with liquid. Beat whites with cream of tartar until stiff peaks form. Fold the batter into the whites, being careful not to beat. Pour into 9" ungreased tube pan. Bake until done (about 1 hour). Invert cake to cool.

**CHARLOTTE'S CHOCOLATE CAKE

Exchanges per serving: 1 = 1 bread, 1 fat, 1/4 fruit.
Calories per serving: 130   Yield: 9 servings

1/3 cup diet margarine, softened
Non-nutritive sweetener equivalent to 1/4 cup brown sugar
1/4 cup (1 medium) egg
Non-nutritive sweetener equivalent to 1/3 cup sugar
1 1/3 cups flour
3 tablespoons unsweetened cocoa
2 teaspoons baking powder
1/2 teaspoon baking soda
1/2 cup skim milk
1/2 teaspoon vanilla extract
1/2 teaspoon almond extract
2 tablespoons nuts, chopped fine

Preheat oven to 350°. Mix margarine, brown sugar substitute, egg and regular sugar substitute. Beat at high speed two minutes, scraping bowl occasionally. Add flour, cocoa, baking powder, baking soda, skim milk, and extracts and blend at low speed about 2 minutes (batter will be thick). Spread batter into an 8" layer pan which has been well greased and sprinkle with nuts. Bake until tester inserted in center comes out clean.

**GINGERBREAD

Exchanges per serving: 1 = 1 1/2 bread, 1/2 fat.
Calories per serving: 125   Yield: 8 servings

4 tablespoons diet margarine
2 tablespoons molasses
1/2 teaspoon ginger
1/4 teaspoon cinnamon
1/4 teaspoon salt

1 1/2 cups plus 1 tablespoon
  boiling water
1 cup rye flour
1/8 teaspoon baking powder
4 teaspoons baking soda

Preheat oven to 400°. Measure margarine, molasses, ginger, cinnamon, and salt into bowl; add boiling water. Sift flour, baking powder, and baking soda into mixture and beat. Pour into greased oblong pan. Bake 30 minutes.

**CHOCOLATE CHIFFON CAKE WITH RUM

Exchanges per serving: 1 1/2" slice = 2 bread, 3 fat, 1/2 meat.
Calories per serving: 175   Yield: 12 servings

2 cups (8 medium) eggs
1/2 cup cocoa
3/4 cup boiling water
Non-nutritive sweetener
  equivalent to 1 3/4 cups
  sugar

1 1/2 teaspoons baking soda
1 3/4 cups flour
1/2 cup soy oil
2 tablespoons rum extract
1/2 teaspoon cream of tartar

Preheat oven to 325°. Let eggs reach room temperature then separate them. Combine cocoa and water in small bowl. Stir until smooth; cool. Sift sweetener, baking soda, and flour into large bowl; make well in center and add oil, egg yolks, rum extract, and cocoa mixture. Beat until smooth. Add cream of tartar to the egg whites and beat very stiff. Pour batter over whites and gently fold into whites until just blended. Bake in ungreased bundt pan (or 10" tube pan) until straw inserted comes out clean. Cool cake completely, then remove from pan. Serve either plain or top with nondairy whipping cream.

**NO CRUST CHEESECAKE

Exchanges per serving: 1" x 1/2" = 2 fat, 1/2 meat.
Calories per serving: 140   Yield: 24 servings

2 cups nonfat cottage cheese
2 cups creamed cheese
Non-nutritive sweetener
  equivalent to 1 1/2 cups
  sugar
3/4 cup (3 medium) eggs
1 1/2 tablespoons lemon juice

1 teaspoon vanilla extract
1/2 cup diet margarine, melted
1 1/2 tablespoons arrowroot
  powder
3 tablespoons flour
2 cups artificial sour cream

Preheat oven to 325°. Cream the cheeses together gradually adding sweetener, beating after each addition. Add eggs, beat well; add lemon juice, vanilla extract, and margarine. Mix arrowroot and flour with enough sour cream to make a smooth paste. Add paste and remaining sour cream; blend thoroughly. Pour into greased 9" spring pan. Bake 1 hour or longer until firm, then turn off oven. Let cake remain in oven 2 hours or longer. Place in refrigerator overnight. Serve cold.

**LORENE'S CHEESECAKE

Exchanges per serving: 1" x 1/2" piece = 1 1/2 fat, 3/4 meat.
Calories per serving: 141

Yield: 24 servings

3/4 cup diet margarine
Non-nutritive sweetener equivalent to 1 1/4 cups sugar
1 cup (4 medium) eggs
2 cups creamed low-calorie cottage cheese
3 tablespoons arrowroot powder

2 cups low-calorie cream cheese (2 8-ounce packages)
6 level tablespoons flour
1 cup imitation sour cream
1/2 teaspoon vanilla extract
1/2 teaspoon lemon juice
1 cup artificially sweetened crushed pineapple

Preheat oven to 325°. Cream first two ingredients; add eggs, cottage cheese, arrowroot, cream cheese and beat well after each addition; add flour, sour cream, vanilla extract, lemon juice, and crushed pineapple, stirring well. Place in spring pan. Bake 2 hours. When baked, the dough will rise over edge but will not run out. Leave in oven for 2 hours with heat off, then leave in refrigerator overnight.

**ORANGE CAKE

Exchanges per serving: 1 = 1 bread, 1 fat, 1/2 meat.
Calories per serving: 150

Yield: 10 servings

1 cup flour
1 1/2 teaspoons baking powder
1/2 teaspoon salt
1/4 cup oil
1 cup (4 medium) eggs, separated

1/2 cup unsweetened frozen orange juice concentrate
Non-nutritive sweetener equivalent to 1 1/2 cups sugar
1/4 teaspoon cream of tartar

Preheat oven to 350°. Sift flour, baking powder, and salt together. Set aside one yolk. Add, in order, oil, egg yolks, orange juice, and sweetener. Beat until smooth. Add cream of tartar to whites of eggs and beat until stiff. Add egg yolk mixture to whites and fold in gently until blended. Do not overmix. Pour into 9" tube pan and bake 35 minutes.

**PAM'S QUICK LAYER CAKE

Exchanges per serving: 1 1/2" slice = 1 bread, 1 1/2 fat, 1/2 meat.
1/8 skim milk.

Calories per serving: 175

Yield: 12 servings

Non-nutritive sweetener
  equivalent to 1 cup sugar
1/16 teaspoon salt
2 cups flour
3 teaspoons baking powder
1/3 cup diet margarine

1/4 cup (1 medium) egg
3/4 cup skim milk
1/2 teaspoon vanilla extract
1/2 teaspoon almond extract
1 cup pecans, chopped extra
  fine

Preheat oven to 375°. Sift sweetener, salt, flour, and baking powder
three or four times. Cut in margarine with pastry blender or knife until
mixture resembles cornmeal. Beat egg until lemon-colored and thick;
then add skim milk and extracts. Add to first mixture gradually. Add
nuts and stir well. Pour into two 8" layer pans which have been well
greased. Bake about 25 minutes. Cool; remove cake from pans. Cool
further on wire rack.

**SOUTHERN HOSPITALITY CAKE

Exchanges per serving: 1 = 1 bread, 2 fat, 1/2 fruit.
Calories per serving: 175

Yield: 9 servings

1/3 cup diet margarine, softened
Non-nutritive sweetener
  equivalent to 3/4 cup sugar
1/4 cup (1 medium) egg
1 1/3 cups flour
1 teaspoon baking powder

1/2 teaspoon baking soda
1/2 teaspoon orange extract
2/3 cup fresh orange juice
1/3 cup raisins
2 tablespoons nuts, chopped
  fine

Preheat oven to 350°. Combine margarine, sweetener, and egg and
beat 2 minutes on high speed of mixer. Scrape bowl occasionally. Add
flour, baking powder, baking soda, orange extract, and juice. Blend at
low speed about 2 minutes (batter will be fairly thick). Then stir in
raisins and spread batter in an 8" layer pan which has been well
greased. Sprinkle nuts on top. Bake until golden brown (about 1/2
hour).

**FAMILY FAVORITE CAKE

Exchanges per serving: 1 1/2" slice = 1 bread, 1 1/2 fat, 1/4 meat, 1/8
skim milk.

Calories per serving: 195

Yield: 15 servings

3/4 cup diet margarine
Non-nutritive sweetener
  equivalent to 1 1/2 cups
  sugar
4 teaspoons baking powder
1/2 teaspoon salt

3 cups flour
1 cup skim milk
1 teaspoon almond extract
3/4 cup (4-5 medium) egg
  whites

Preheat oven to 375°. Cream margarine and sweetener. Sift baking powder, salt, and flour, then add alternately with skim milk to creamed mixture. Add almond extract, and beat stiff and fold in whites. Pour into two well-greased 9" layer pans. Bake about 30 minutes. Cool a few minutes, then remove cake from pans and cool further on wire rack.

**ORANGE CHIFFON CAKE

Exchanges per serving: 1 1/2" slice = 2 bread, 1 fat, 1/8 skim milk.
Calories per serving: 135   Yield: 16 servings

2 cups (about 8) eggs, separated
2 1/4 cups flour, sifted
3 teaspoons baking powder
1 teaspoon salt
3 tablespoons orange peel, grated fine
1/2 cup salad oil

Non-nutritive sweetener equivalent to 1 1/2 cups sugar
Artificial sweetener equivalent to 1/4 cup sugar added to 3/4 cup orange juice
1/2 teaspoon cream of tartar

Preheat oven to 325°. Set aside 3 egg yolks and cover remaining eggs until they are room temperature. (Refrigerate the 3 yolks for other use.) Add cream of tartar to egg whites and beat until they stand in peaks (stiffer than for meringue). Sift dry ingredients, make a well in center, add salad oil, egg yolks, peel, and juice-sweetener mixture. Stir to blend. Beat one minute at medium speed. Add yolk-orange mixture to whites slowly, folding these together until smooth and completely mixed. Pour into a 2" x 9" x 9" cake pan which has first been rinsed and excess water shaken out. Bake until cake is pale golden brown and a cake tester comes out clean (about 1/2 hour or a little more). Invert pan and cool. When cake pan is cool enough to handle (but not cold) run a knife around edges of pan, then with fingertips carefully take cake away from edges, lifting slightly to loosen bottom. Cool on rack. Cut into serving pieces.

**EASY SPONGE CAKE

Exchanges per serving: 1 = 1 bread, 1/2 meat.
Calories per serving: 110   Yield: 8 servings

1 cup (4 medium) eggs, separated
Non-nutritive sweetener equivalent to 1 cup sugar
1 cup flour

1 teaspoon baking powder
1/2 teaspoon vanilla
or
1/2 teaspoon lemon juice

Preheat oven to 300°. Beat egg whites very stiff; beat yolks very lightly. Add half the sweetener to whites, the rest to yolks. Put together and beat hard; sift flour with baking powder and fold in. Add vanilla or lemon juice. Place in angel tin and bake 40 minutes.

**CUPCAKES

Exchanges per serving: 1 cupcake = 3/4 bread, 1 1/2 fat.
Calories per serving: 140   Yield: 12 cupcakes

1 1/2 cups flour
1 1/2 teaspoons baking pow-
    der
1/2 teaspoon salt
1/4 teaspoon baking soda
1/2 teaspoon cinnamon
1/2 teaspoon allspice

1/2 teaspoon nutmeg
1/4 teaspoon ground cloves
1/2 cup diet margarine
1/2 cup (2 medium) eggs
Non-nutritive sweetener
    equivalent to 2/3 cup sugar
1/2 cup white raisins

1/2 cup cold water

Preheat oven to 350°. Combine flour, baking powder, salt, baking
soda, cinnamon, allspice, nutmeg, and cloves; cut in margarine until
size of small peas. Add remaining ingredients and mix until all first
mixture is moistened. Fill 12 paper baking cups about 1/2 full and bake
until tester inserted in center comes out clean.

**FRUIT CRISP

Exchanges per serving: 1 = 1/2 bread, 1/2 fat, 1 1/2 fruit.
Calories per serving: 115   Yield: 6 servings

4 cups fruit, peeled and sliced
    thin (apples, peaches, apri-
    cots)
Non-nutritive sweetener
    equivalent to 2/3 cup sugar
1 teaspoon fresh lemon juice
1/2 cup quick-cooking rolled
    oats

Non-nutritive sweetener
    equivalent to 2 tablespoons
    brown sugar
1 tablespoon arrowroot pow-
    der
1/4 teaspoon allspice
2 tablespoons diet margarine

Preheat oven to 350°. Combine fruit with sweetener equivalent to 1/3
cup regular sugar and juice. Place in casserole. Combine oats, brown
sugar substitute, arrowroot, allspice and rest of regular sugar substitute. Cut in margarine until crumbly, then sprinkle evenly over fruit.
Bake about 1 hour, or until tender. Serve hot or cold.

***LOU'S LIGHT CAKE

Exchanges per serving: 1 = 2 fat, 2 bread.
Calories per serving: 215   Yield: 10 servings

2/3 cup diet margarine
Non-nutritive sweetener
    equivalent to 2 cups sugar
2 teaspoons vanilla extract
2 teaspoons boiling water
1 1/2 cups cold water

3 1/2 cups sifted flour
1/2 teaspoon salt
4 teaspoons baking powder
3/4 cup (4-5 medium) egg
    whites

Preheat oven to 350°. Cream margarine and sweetener, add vanilla and boiling water and blend thoroughly. Add cold water and beat 1 minute. Sift flour and salt four times, then add bit by bit alternating with small amounts of the water mixture, beating well after each addition. Sift baking powder over top of batter and fold in gently with stiffly beaten egg whites. Bake in two 10-inch pans which have been well greased and floured, until done.

***LU'S CHIFFON CAKE

Exchanges per serving: 1 = 1 1/2 bread, 2 fat, 1/2 meat.
Calories per serving: 215   Yield: 12 servings

1 teaspoon salt
2 1/4 cups flour, sifted
3 teaspoons baking powder
1/2 cup salad oil
1 cup (4 medium) eggs, separated
1/2 cup water

Non-nutritive sweetener equivalent to 1 1/2 cups sugar
2 teaspoons lemon rind, grated
1 teaspoon vanilla extract
1/2 teaspoon cream of tartar

Preheat oven to 325°. Sift salt, flour, and baking powder. Add oil, well-beaten egg yolks, water, sweetener, rind, and vanilla extract. Beat until smooth. Beat egg whites until stiff, add cream of tartar and beat until very stiff peaks form. Gently fold the batter into egg whites until just blended (but do not stir). Place in ungreased 9" tube pan. Bake until done (about 1 hour). Invert cake to cool.

****MARGARET'S POUND CAKE

Exchanges per serving: 1 1/2" slice = 1 bread, 1 fat, 1/2 meat.
Calories per serving: 350   Yield: 15 servings

1 teaspoon salt
4 cups flour
1/2 teaspoon cream of tartar
2 cups diet margarine
1/2 teaspoon allspice

Non-nutritive sweetener equivalent to 2 cups sugar
2 cups (8 medium) eggs
1 teaspoon vanilla extract

Preheat oven to 325°. Sift salt, flour, and cream of tartar, and set aside. Cream margarine until fluffy, then add sweetener gradually and continue to cream until very fluffy. Beat in eggs 1/4 cup at a time, add vanilla extract and allspice. Beat well, then add flour mixture a little at a time until well mixed. Turn batter into greased and lightly floured bundt pan (or 2 bread pans). Bake 1 1/4 to 1 1/2 hours for bundt cake or 1 hour for loaf cakes. Cool in pans; then turn out on wire rack and cool completely. May be sprinkled with substitute for confectioners' sugar.

***STRAWBERRY SHORTCAKE

Exchanges per serving: 1 cake = 2 bread, 2 fat.
1/2 cup berries = 1/2 fruit.

Calories per serving: 1 cake: 220
berries: 20 Yield: 6 servings

2 cups flour
Non-nutritive sweetener
equivalent to 1 tablespoon
sugar
1/2 teaspoon salt
3 teaspoons baking powder
4 tablespoons diet margarine

1/2 cup water
1 quart strawberries (or other
fruit) sweetened with equivalent to 1 teaspoon sugar
1 cup nonfat cream, whipped
with equivalent to 1 tea-
spoon sugar

Preheat oven to 475°. Sift flour, sweetener, salt, and baking powder; add margarine and mix thoroughly with steel fork. Add water to make dough soft. Roll out on floured board until about 1/2" thick. Cut with large biscuit cutter dipped in flour, or half fill large greased muffin rings which have been placed on baking pan. Bake 10-12 minutes. Split while hot, butter, and fill with crushed sweetened berries. Put on tops and cover with strawberries and sweetened whipped cream. For nonfat whipping cream, check the label for calorie content of cream used.

*CAKE FILLING

Exchanges per serving: 1 tablespoon = trace meat.
Calories per serving: 10 (plus calories for
frosting) Yield: 1 1/2 cups

1 recipe Lemon Frosting (see
recipe)
1 cup nonfat cottage cheese,
drained and sieved

1 1/2 teaspoons unflavored
gelatin
2 tablespoons water

To Lemon Frosting, add cottage cheese and beat until smooth. Add gelatin to water and dissolve over boiling water (about 5 minutes). Blend carefully and use at once.

*CREAMY FROSTING

Exchanges per serving: 1 tablespoon = trace fat, trace meat.
Calories per serving: 15 Yield: 1/2 cup

1/2 cup nonfat cottage cheese,
sieved
1/8 teaspoon salt
1/2 tablespoon diet margarine, melted

Non-nutritive sweetener
equivalent to 1/2 cup sugar
1 teaspoon almond or vanilla
extract

Mix all ingredients. Beat until smooth. Spread on cake. (Frosts one 10" cake.)

*LEMON FROSTING

Exchanges per serving: 1 tablespoon = 1/4 skim milk.
Calories per serving: 20   Yield: 1/3 cup

2 tablespoons nonfat dry milk
1 1/2 teaspoons lemon juice
Non-nutritive sweetener equivalent to 2 tablespoons sugar

1 teaspoon vanilla
2 tablespoons water
1/2 teaspoon unflavored gelatin

Combine all ingredients except water and gelatin. Dissolve 1/2 teaspoon gelatin and 2 tablespoons water over hot water. Beat rest of ingredients at high speed of electric mixer about 15 minutes. Add gelatin gradually. Continue beating until frosting stands in peaks. Use right away.

*LOW-CALORIE FROSTING

Exchanges per serving: 1 tablespoon = 3/4 fat.
Calories per serving: 30   Yield: 3 tablespoons

2 tablespoons cream cheese
1 teaspoon skim milk
Non-nutritive sweetener equivalent to 2 tablespoons powdered sugar

1/8 teaspoon salt
1/4 teaspoon vanilla extract
1/16 teaspoon food coloring

Cream cheese and skim milk thoroughly. Add sweetener, salt, and vanilla extract. Blend well. Add coloring last, using green for St. Patrick's Day, red for Christmas, etc.

COOKIES

*BUTTERSCOTCH SQUARES

Exchanges per serving: 1 square = 1/2 fat.
Calories per serving: 25

Yield: 70 squares

1/2 cup diet margarine
Non-nutritive sweetener equivalent to 2 cups brown sugar

1/2 cup (2 medium) eggs
1 1/2 cups flour
2 teaspoons baking powder
1 teaspoon vanilla extract

1/2 cup walnuts, chopped

Preheat oven to 350°. Cook margarine and sweetener together until smooth. Cool to lukewarm. Add eggs and beat well. Add flour, baking powder, vanilla, and walnuts. Spread in 9" x 12" x 2" pan which has been lightly greased. Bake 1/2 hour. Cut in squares 1 1/4" x 1 1/4". Sprinkle with non-nutritive granulated sugar. Cool.

*MARY'S CHOCOLATE CHIP COOKIES

Exchanges per serving: 1 cookie = 1/4 bread, 3/4 fat.
Calories per serving: 50

Yield: 3 dozen cookies

1/4 teaspoon salt
1/2 teaspoon baking soda
1 cup flour, sifted
1/2 cup diet margarine
Non-nutritive sweetener equivalent to 2/3 cup plus 4 teaspoons sugar

1/2 teaspoon vanilla extract
1/4 cup (1 medium) egg, beaten
1/2 cup semisweet chocolate, shaved fine

Preheat oven to 375°. Sift salt, baking soda, and flour together. Cream margarine and add sweetener, vanilla, and egg, blending well. Add flour mixture. Beat well; stir in chocolate. Drop by level spoonsful onto a baking sheet which has been lightly greased. Bake about 10 minutes.

*ANGEL'S KISS

Exchanges per serving: 1 kiss = 1/8 fat, 1/8 meat.
Calories per serving: 15

Yield: 3 dozen kisses

Non-nutritive sweetener equivalent to 1 1/2 cups confectioners' sugar
1 1/2 cups (9 medium) egg yolks, lightly beaten

1/2 cup blanched almonds, finely cut
1 teaspoon instant diet tea mix
1 teaspoon almond extract

Preheat oven to 325°. Beat sweetener into yolks; add almonds, tea mix, and almond extract. (Mixture will be runny.) Line muffin pans with paper baking cups and fill each half full. Bake until golden brown; remove cups while warm. Cool on wire rack.

*BUTTERMILK OAT COOKIES

Exchanges per serving: 1 square = 1/4 bread, 1/4 fat.
Calories per serving: 25   Yield: 2 1/2 dozen cookies

1 cup flour
1/2 cup rolled oats, uncooked
1/4 teaspoon baking soda
1/2 teaspoon salt

Non-nutritive sweetener
  equivalent to 3 tablespoons
  sugar
1/4 cup buttermilk
1/4 cup diet margarine, or
  butter, melted

Preheat oven to 400°. Sift flour, oats, baking soda, and salt. Add sweetener to buttermilk, then stir this and margarine into flour mixture until dry ingredients are moistened. Knead dough lightly on well-floured board for a few moments, then roll thin. Cut into 2" x 2" squares. Bake on ungreased cookie sheet until brown (10-12 minutes).

*BROWNIES

Exchanges per serving: 1 brownie = 1/4 bread, 1 fat.
Calories per serving: 65   Yield: 5 dozen brownies

1 cup diet margarine
2 squares unsweetened chocolate
2 cups flour
1 teaspoon salt
1 teaspoon baking soda

Non-nutritive sweetener
  equivalent to 5 cups sugar
1 cup (4 medium) eggs, well
  beaten
4 teaspoons vanilla extract
1/2 cup chopped nuts

Preheat oven to 325°. Melt margarine and chocolate over low heat; then remove. Sift together flour, salt, and baking soda. Add sweetener, eggs, and vanilla extract and stir into dry ingredients until well blended; stir in nuts. Pour into 8" square pan which has been well greased. Bake 20 minutes. Cool. Cut into squares.

*TASTY DIET BROWNIES

Exchanges per serving: 1 brownie = 1/4 bread, 1 fat.
Calories per serving: 65   Yield: 16 brownies

2/3 cup flour, sifted
1/2 teaspoon baking powder
1/4 teaspoon salt
1 ounce unsweetened chocolate (1 square)
1/4 cup (1 medium) egg

1/2 cup dietetic maple topping
Non-nutritive sweetener
  equivalent to 2 teaspoons
  sugar
1/3 cup chopped walnuts
1/2 teaspoon vanilla extract

Preheat oven to 350°. Measure flour, add baking powder and salt and sift again. Melt chocolate over hot water. Beat egg one minute, add topping and sweetener and beat two more minutes, then add melted chocolate and blend. Add flour and stir (do not beat) until smooth. Add walnuts and vanilla extract. Spread batter 1/2" to 3/4" thick in 8" square pan (or 9" pie tin). Bake 40 minutes.

*SPICY COOKIES

Exchanges per serving: 1 cookie = 1/8 bread, 1 fat.
Calories per serving: 55   Yield: 24 cookies

1/3 cup diet margarine
1 cup flour
1/4 teaspoon baking powder
1/4 teaspoon salt
2 tablespoons cocoa

1 tablespoon water
Non-nutritive sweetener
  equivalent to 1/3 cup sugar
1/2 teaspoon cinnamon
1/2 teaspoon nutmeg

1 teaspoon vanilla extract

Preheat oven to 375°. Cream margarine until light and nearly cream colored. Sift flour, baking powder, salt, and cocoa together and blend into margarine until smooth. Mix water, sweetener, cinnamon, nutmeg, and vanilla extract; add to flour-margarine mixture and mix until smooth (dough will be stiff). Shape into balls about 3/4" round. Place on cookie sheet; flatten with blade of knife dipped into cold water. Bake until done (about 15 minutes). Remove from tray and cool.

*CHOCOLATE COOKIES

Exchanges per serving: 1 cookie, 2" diameter = trace bread, trace
                       meat.
Calories per serving: 22   Yield: 2 1/2 dozen cookies

1/4 cup (1 medium) egg, separated
Non-nutritive sweetener
  equivalent to 1/3 cup sugar
2 teaspoons unsweetened fruit
  liquid, any kind

1 cup flour
1 teaspoon baking powder
1/4 teaspoon salt
1/2 cup unsweetened chocolate topping
1/4 teaspoon cream of tartar

Preheat oven to 325°. Mix egg yolks, sweetener, and fruit liquid together in large bowl. Beat with electric mixer until light and fluffy (about 10-12 minutes). Meanwhile sift flour, baking powder, and salt together 3 times. Add chocolate topping to first mixture and beat until mixed thoroughly. Beat egg whites with cream of tartar until they stand in soft peaks. Very carefully fold dry ingredients into chocolate topping mix. Fold beaten egg whites into this mixture and then drop by teaspoonful onto lightly greased cookie sheet. Bake about 10 minutes or until cookie springs back when lightly touched. Remove cookies to wire rack to cool, with spatula.

*MARY'S THUMBPRINTS

Exchanges per serving: 1 cookie = 1/4 fat.
Calories per serving: 20   Yield: 4 dozen cookies

1/2 cup diet margarine
Non-nutritive sweetener
  equivalent to 1/4 cup sugar
1/4 cup (1 medium) egg, separated
1 tablespoon orange rind

1 1/2 teaspoons lemon rind
1/2 teaspoon vanilla extract
1 tablespoon lemon juice
1 tablespoon orange juice
1 cup flour
1 teaspoon salt

1/2 cup nuts, finely chopped

Preheat oven to 350°. Mix together everything except the egg whites
and nuts and roll into small balls. Beat the egg whites stiff and spread
the nuts out on a piece of waxed paper. Roll each ball in egg white, then
in the nuts, and make a thumbprint in each. Bake 12 minutes. Cool.
When cooled, fill each thumbprint with diet jelly.

*SPICY APPLESAUCE COOKIES

Exchanges per serving: 1 cookie, 2" diameter = 1 bread, 1 fruit.
Calories per serving: 20   Yield: 3 1/2 dozen cookies

1 cup flour
1/3 cup nonfat dry milk solids
1 teaspoon baking powder
1/2 teaspoon cinnamon
1/4 teaspoon nutmeg
1/4 teaspoon cloves
1/8 teaspoon salt
1/2 cup (2 medium) eggs
Non-nutritive sweetener
  equivalent to 8 teaspoons
  sugar

3 tablespoons unsweetened
  fruit liquid (any fruit)
1/2 cup unsweetened ap-
  plesauce
10 almonds, blanched and cut
  in quarters

Preheat oven to 325°. Sift dry ingredients together three times; mix
eggs, sweetener, and fruit liquid. Beat at top speed of mixer until fluffy
and thick (about 10 minutes). Decrease speed. Add applesauce and beat
three minutes; carefully fold in dry ingredients. Drop by teaspoonsful
onto lightly greased cookie sheet. Place 1/4 almond on each cookie.
Bake about 10 minutes. Cookie will spring back at light touch when
done. (These may be placed under broiler to give deeper finish.)

*COCONUT FRUIT COOKIES

Exchanges per serving: 1 cookie = 1/2 bread, 1/4 fat.
Calories per serving: 45   Yield: 3 dozen cookies

1 1/2 cups flour
1 teaspoon baking powder
1/4 teaspoon baking soda
1/4 teaspoon salt
1/3 cup diet margarine
1/3 cup flaked coconut
1/4 cup (1 medium) egg

1/2 cup unsweetened fruit
juice
2 teaspoons orange or lemon
peel, grated
Non-nutritive sweetener
equivalent to 1/3 cup sugar
1 teaspoon almond (or vanilla)
extract

Preheat oven to 400°. Combine flour, baking powder, baking soda, and salt, then cut in margarine until consistency of peas. Stir in coconut then add remaining ingredients all at once. Stir with fork until dough holds together. Drop about 2 inches apart by teaspoonsful onto an ungreased cookie sheet. Bake until light golden brown (about 10 minutes).

*YUMMY PEANUT BUTTER COOKIES

Exchanges per serving: 1 cookie = 1/4 bread, 1/4 meat.
Calories per serving: 34   Yield: 1 1/2 dozen cookies

1/3 cup flour
1/4 teaspoon baking soda
1/4 teaspoon baking powder
1/4 cup diet margarine
4 tablespoons peanut butter
Non-nutritive sweetener
equivalent to 1 tablespoon
brown sugar

Non-nutritive sweetener
equivalent to 1/2 cup regular sugar
1/4 cup (1 medium) egg, well
beaten

Preheat oven to 375°. Grease cookie sheet lightly. Sift flour, baking soda, and baking powder. Work margarine and peanut butter with spoon until creamy, then gradually add brown sugar substitute, continuing to work until light. Add regular sugar substitute and egg and beat well. Mix in dry ingredients thoroughly. Drop by teaspoonsful onto lightly greased heavy-duty aluminum foil, then flatten with tines of fork. Bake until done (about 8-10 minutes).

*CHOCOLATE CHIP COOKIES

Exchanges per serving: 1 cookie = 1 fat.
Calories per serving: 45

1 1/2 cups diet margarine, softened
Non-nutritive sweetener equivalent to 3/4 cup sugar
2 tablespoons water
1/2 teaspoon vanilla extract
1/4 cup (1 medium) egg, beaten

1 cup, plus 2 tablespoons all-purpose flour
1/2 teaspoon baking soda
1/2 teaspoon salt
1/2 cup unsweetened chocolate bits
1/2 cup chopped nuts (optional)

Preheat oven to 375°. Cream margarine, mix in sweetener, water, and vanilla extract. To this mixture add the beaten egg. Sift flour, baking soda, and salt together; stir into mixture. Mix in chocolate bits and nuts. Drop by spoon onto greased cookie sheet. Bake from 10-12 minutes.

*CREAM CHEESE-COCONUT DELIGHT

Exchanges per serving: 1 cookie = 2 fat.
Calories per serving: 90   Yield: 2 dozen cookies

2 ounces cream cheese
Non-nutritive sweetener equivalent to 1/2 cup sugar
1 teaspoon orange rind, grated
1 teaspoon lemon rind, grated

2 teaspoons walnuts, chopped fine
1/2 cup coconut, shredded and toasted

Work cream cheese with spoon until light and fluffy. Thoroughly mix sweetener, both grated rinds, and nuts. Add to cheese. Form in 1" balls. Roll in toasted coconut and refrigerate.

**JOAN'S PEANUT BUTTER COOKIES

Exchanges per serving: 5 cookies = 1/2 bread, 1 fat, 1/2 meat.
Calories per serving: 116   Yield: 4 dozen cookies

1/4 cup diet margarine
Non-nutritive sweetener equivalent to 1 cup sugar
1/2 cup peanut butter, softened

1/4 cup (1 medium) egg
1/3 cup skim milk
1 teaspoon vanilla extract
1 cup flour
1/4 teaspoon salt
1 teaspoon baking powder

Preheat oven to 375°. Combine margarine, sweetener, peanut butter, and blend well. Combine egg, milk, and vanilla extract, and add to first mixture. Sift flour, salt, and baking powder together and add, blending well. Drop by spoonsful onto cookie sheet which has been greased (or onto heavy-duty aluminum foil). Flatten with tines of fork dipped in water. Bake 10 minutes.

*REFRIGERATED COCONUT FRUIT COOKIES

Exchanges per serving: 1 cookie = 1/4 bread, 1/4 fat.
Calories per serving: 30   Yield: 2 1/2 dozen cookies

Non-nutritive sweetener equivalent to 1/2 cup sugar
1/4 cup unsweetened fruit juice
1 teaspoon vanilla extract

1/4 teaspoon baking powder
1/4 teaspoon salt
1 cup flour
1/4 cup diet margarine
2 tablespoons coconut

Combine sweetener, juice, and vanilla extract. Sift baking powder, salt, and flour and then cut the margarine into this. Add the liquid ingredients. After these are well mixed, work in coconut. Make dough into a roll about 2" diameter and place in waxed paper in refrigerator until well chilled and firm. Slice into 2 1/2 dozen cookies and place on ungreased cookie sheet. Preheat oven to 400°. Bake 10 minutes.

*CRISP APPLESAUCE COOKIES

Exchanges per serving: 1 cookie = 1/4 bread, 1/4 fat, 1/4 fruit.
Calories per cookie: 40   Yield: 4 dozen cookies

1 2/3 cups flour, sifted
1 teaspoon cinnamon
1/4 teaspoon nutmeg
1/4 teaspoon cloves
1/2 teaspoon allspice
1/2 teaspoon salt
1 teaspoon baking soda

1/2 cup diet margarine
Non-nutritive sweetener equivalent to 1 cup sugar
1/4 cup (1 medium) egg
1 cup unsweetened applesauce
1/3 cup white raisins
1 cup whole bran cereal

Preheat oven to 375°. Sift dry ingredients together. Mix margarine, sweetener, and eggs until light and fluffy; then add flour mixture and applesauce alternately. Mix well after each addition. Fold in raisins and cereal and drop by teaspoonsful onto well-greased sheet of heavy-duty aluminum foil about 1" apart. Bake until golden brown (about 15 minutes).

*CHOCOLATE BITES

Exchanges per serving: 1 cookie = 1/2 fat, 1/4 bread.
Calories per serving: 36   Yield: 2 1/2 dozen cookies

1/3 cup diet margarine	2 teaspoons vanilla extract
1/4 cup cocoa	1 cup flour
2 tablespoons liquid sweetener	1/2 teaspoon baking soda
1/2 cup (2 medium) eggs, well beaten	1/2 teaspoon salt

Preheat oven to 325°. Melt margarine, add cocoa, sweetener, eggs, and vanilla extract and stir until blended well. Sift flour, baking soda, and salt together, add, and mix well (batter will be quite dry). Spread on 8" square pan which has been well greased. Bake about 20 minutes. Cool and cut into bites.

*ORANGE COOKIES WITH NUTS

Exchanges per serving: 1 cookie = 1/4 bread, 1/2 fat.
Calories per serving: 40   Yield: 2 1/2 dozen cookies

1/2 cup frozen unsweetened orange juice concentrate	1 cup flour
1/4 cup (1 medium) egg	1/4 teaspoon salt
1/4 cup diet margarine	1/4 teaspoon baking powder
Non-nutritive sweetener equivalent to 1 cup sugar	1 teaspoon vanilla extract
	1/2 cup pecans, chopped fine

Preheat oven to 375°. Cream first four ingredients and beat well. Sift flour, salt, and baking powder and add to creamed mixture. Mix gently, until just blended; add vanilla extract and nuts. Drop by teaspoonsful onto lightly greased heavy-duty aluminum foil, and bake until lightly browned (about 15 minutes).

*RICE FLOUR COOKIES

Exchanges per serving: 1 cookie = 1/4 bread, 1/4 fat.
Calories per serving: 27   Yield: 2 dozen cookies

3/4 cup diet margarine	1/2 teaspoon almond extract
Non-nutritive sweetener equivalent to 1 1/2 cups sugar	1 teaspoon orange or lemon extract
1/2 cup (2 medium) eggs	2 1/2 cups rice flour
1/2 teaspoon vanilla extract	1 teaspoon cream of tartar
	1 teaspoon baking soda

Preheat oven to 375°. Cream margarine and sweetener; add eggs and extracts. Sift flour, cream of tartar, and baking soda; mix all ingredients well, then roll in small balls. Place on greased cookie sheet (or on heavy-duty aluminum foil) and flatten with tines of fork. Bake until brown (10 minutes).

*ORANGE OR LEMON PEEL COOKIES

Exchanges per serving: 1 cookie = 1/2 bread, 1 fat.
Calories per serving: 79

Yield: 4 dozen cookies

1/2 cup diet margarine
Non-nutritive sweetener equivalent to 1/2 cup sugar
1/3 cup hot water
1 teaspoon orange extract
1 teaspoon vanilla extract

2 cups flour
1 teaspoon baking powder
1/2 teaspoon salt
3/4 cup pecans, chopped fine
1 tablespoon orange or lemon peel, finely grated

Cream first five ingredients, then sift together and add flour, baking powder, and salt. Blend in pecans and orange or lemon peel until mixture is smooth. Shape dough into roll about 2" x 4". Wrap in waxed paper; chill well in refrigerator. Cut roll into 48 cookies; place on lightly greased heavy-duty aluminum foil. Preheat oven to 400°; bake until brown around edges, about 12-15 minutes.

*OATMEAL COOKIES

Exchanges per serving: 1 cookie = 1/4 bread, 1/4 fat, 1/4 fruit.
Calories per serving: 35

Yield: 4 dozen cookies

1 1/2 cups quick-cooking oatmeal, uncooked
2/3 cup diet margarine, melted
1/2 cup (2 medium) eggs, beaten
Non-nutritive sweetener equivalent to 1 1/2 cups sugar

1 1/2 cups flour, sifted
2 teaspoons baking powder
1/2 teaspoon salt
1/2 cup skim milk
1 teaspoon vanilla extract
1/4 cup raisins

Preheat oven to 400°. Measure oatmeal into bowl, stir in melted margarine and mix well. Stir in eggs and sweetener, then add flour, baking powder, and salt, alternating with the combined milk and vanilla. Add raisins. Drop onto cookie sheet from level teaspoonsful and bake until golden brown (about 10-15 minutes).

*FRUIT COOKIES

Exchanges per serving: 1 cookie = 1/3 bread, 1/2 fat, 1/4 fruit.
Calories per serving: 56   Yield: 20 cookies

1/2 cup flour
1/8 teaspoon cloves
1/4 teaspoon nutmeg
1 teaspoon cinnamon
1/4 teaspoon salt
1/2 teaspoon baking soda
1/2 cup raisins

1/2 cup rolled oats, uncooked
1/2 cup unsweetened cranberry sauce
1/2 cup diet margarine, melted
1/4 cup (1 medium) egg
1 teaspoon vanilla extract

Preheat oven to 375°. Sift flour, cloves, nutmeg, cinnamon, salt, and baking soda together, then add raisins and oats. Combine cranberry sauce, margarine, egg, and vanilla extract. Stir into dry ingredients until they are moistened. Using lightly greased cookie sheet, drop by teaspoonsful and bake 10-12 minutes.

*MACAROONS

Exchanges per serving: 1 macaroon = 1/2 fat.
Calories per serving: 24   Yield: 3 1/2 dozen macaroons

1/4 cup (1 medium) egg, separated
Non-nutritive sweetener equivalent to 1 cup sugar

2 cups cornflakes
1 cup shredded coconut
1/2 cup chopped pecans (optional)
1/2 teaspoon almond extract

Beat egg whites until stiff but not dry. Fold in sweetener, then add cornflakes, coconut, chopped pecans, and almond extract. Drop from teaspoon onto greased baking sheet and bake at 350° for about 12 minutes. Remove at once from baking sheet.

*GRANDMA'S COOKIES

Exchanges per serving: 1 cookie = 1/2 bread, 1 fat.
Calories per serving: 85   Yield: 2 dozen cookies

2/3 cup diet margarine
Non-nutritive sweetener equivalent to 3/4 cup sugar
1 teaspoon vanilla extract
1/4 cup (1 medium) egg

4 teaspoons milk
2 cups all-purpose flour, sifted
1 1/2 teaspoons baking powder
1/4 teaspoon salt

Thoroughly cream margarine, sweetener, and vanilla extract. Add egg and beat until light and fluffy; then stir in milk. Sift flour, baking powder, and salt together: blend into creamed mixture. Divide dough in half and chill 1 hour. Roll half of the dough at a time. (Keep balance chilled for easier rolling.) On lightly floured surface, roll dough to about 1/2" thickness. Cut in desired shapes. Preheat oven to 375° and bake 6-8 minutes. Cool slightly, then remove from pan. Top with unsweetened fruit on each one, if desired.

*PEANUT BUTTER COOKIES

Exchanges per serving: 1 cookie = 1/2 bread, 1/2 meat.
Calories per serving: 71 Yield: 8 cookies

- 8 graham crackers, crushed
- 2 tablespoons peanut butter
- Non-nutritive sweetener equivalent to 1/4 cup sugar
- 1 teaspoon baking powder
- 1/4 cup (3 medium) egg yolks
- 1 teaspoon milk

Preheat oven to 340°. Combine cracker crumbs and peanut butter, then add sweetener and baking powder. Add egg yolks and milk and mix well. Divide into eight 1" cookies and press with fork to flatten. Bake 10 minutes.

**BROWNIES DIVINE

Exchanges per serving: 1 brownie = 1/2 bread, 2 fat.
Calories per serving: 120 Yield: 16 brownies

- 1/2 cup diet margarine
- Non-nutritive sweetener equivalent to 1 1/4 cups sugar
- 1 square unsweetened chocolate
- 1 teaspoon vanilla extract
- 1/2 cup (2 medium) eggs
- 3/4 cup flour
- 1 teaspoon baking powder
- 1/2 cup nuts, chopped

Preheat oven to 350°. Cream margarine and sweetener until light and fluffy. Place chocolate on aluminum foil and melt over boiling water. Stir chocolate into margarine mixture and beat until smooth. Then beat in vanilla and eggs. Sift and stir together flour and baking powder; add nuts, then stir this mixture into first mixture until smooth. Grease a 2" x 8" x 8" pan; spread batter into this. Bake until brownies are shiny, about half an hour. Cool in pan. Cut into 16 pieces and serve cool.

PIES AND PIE CRUSTS

*DIETETIC APPLE CRUNCH

Exchanges per serving: 1 = 1/2 bread, 1/2 fat, 1 fruit.
Calories per serving: 86   Yield: 6 servings

2 slices dry bread
1 tablespoon diet margarine
1/2 teaspoon cinnamon
3/4 cup dietetic maple topping
1/2 teaspoon allspice
3 cups apples, sliced
1 tablespoon lemon juice

Preheat oven to 350°. Make crumbs from bread and toast in oven. Mix toasted crumbs with margarine, cinnamon, and 1/4 teaspoon allspice. Mix apples with lemon juice, maple topping, and rest of allspice. Spread in well-greased shallow baking dish (approximately 8" round). Cover with crumb mixture and bake 45 minutes, or until apple slices are tender. Serve warm.

*ICEBOX CHOCOLATE PIE

Exchanges per serving: 1 = 1/2 bread, 1/3 fat, 1/4 milk.
Calories per serving: 100   Yield: 8 servings

2 tablespoons cocoa
1/8 teaspoon salt
1 1/2 teaspoons arrowroot powder
1/2 cup skim milk, scalded
1/4 cup (1 medium) egg, separated
Non-nutritive sweetener equivalent to 3/4 cup sugar
1/2 cup evaporated milk, beaten
1 teaspoon vanilla
12 graham crackers

Mix cocoa, salt, and arrowroot, then blend in skim milk. Add slightly beaten egg yolk and sweetener. Cook in top of double boiler until thickened. Cool. Beat the egg white, evaporated milk, and vanilla until stiff and fold in. Roll graham crackers into crumbs and use half in 8" pie pan; pour in filling. Use remaining crumbs on top. Put in freezer until firm.

**PEACH PIE FILLING

Exchanges per serving: 1 filling = 1/2 fruit.
                       1 pastry = 1 bread, 1 1/2 fat.

Calories per serving: filling: 20   Yield: 10 servings
                      pastry: 135

2 cups firm, ripe peaches   1/4 teaspoon lemon juice
1/4 tablespoon salt   2 tablespoons diet margarine
1 quart + 1/4 cup water   Pastry for one 10" pie crust
Non-nutritive sweetener
  equivalent to 1/2 cup sugar

Remove peach skins and pits; slice peaches and drop into solution of
salt and 1 quart hot water. Drain. Mix sweetener, 1/4 cup water, and
lemon juice together; pour over peaches. Set in refrigerator until cool.
Place in unbaked 10" crust and dot with margarine. Preheat oven to
325°. Bake peaches until they are tender to the touch of a fork (about
30-40 minutes).

**MARGARET'S GLAZED BERRY TARTS

Exchanges per serving: 1 = 3/4 fruit.
                       1 pastry = 1 bread, 1 1/2 fat.

Calories per serving: filling: 30
                      pastry: 135   Yield: 6 servings

1 envelope unflavored gelatin   Non-nutritive sweetener
1/4 cup cold water   equivalent to 1 1/2 cups
4 cups fresh berries, hulled   sugar
  and washed (strawberries,   3 drops food coloring
  boysenberries, etc.)   2 tablespoons lemon juice
          Pastry for 6 medium tarts

Preheat oven to 425°. Bake tart shells until lightly browned. Remove
from oven and let cool. Soften gelatin in cold water. Sweeten berries
with sweetener and press through strainer until 1 1/2 cups are obtained.
Add coloring and lemon juice and bring to a boil. Remove from heat.
Add softened gelatin and stir to dissolve. Chill until mixture begins to
thicken. Arrange rest of whole berries in baked shells. Cover with
gelatin-berry mixture. May be topped with artificial cream or Low-
Calorie Topping Whip.

**FRUIT SHORTCAKE

Exchanges per serving: 1 shortcake = 1 bread, 1 fat, 1/2 fruit.
Calories per serving: 130   Yield: 6 shortcakes

1 cup flour   1/2 cup skim milk
2 teaspoons baking powder   Non-nutritive sweetener
1/4 teaspoon salt   equivalent to 1 cup sugar
2 tablespoons diet margarine   3 cups fruit, cut up

Preheat oven to 450°. Sift flour, baking powder, and salt together in a small mixing bowl. Cut in margarine until mixture resembles small peas. Combine skim milk and sweetener; add all at once to flour mixture, stirring lightly with a fork until all moistened. Drop by large spoonsful onto a greased sheet of heavy-duty aluminum foil. Bake until golden brown (about 15 minutes). Cool. Split and serve with fruit sweetened to taste with non-nutritive sweetener. Top with Custard Sauce for Shortcakes, if desired.

**BERRY PIE

Exchanges per serving: 1 = 1/2 fruit.

1 crust = 1 bread, 1 1/2 fat.

Calories per serving: filling: 20

crust: 135

Yield: 8 servings

1 quart berries (blueberries, raspberries, etc.)
2 teaspoons lemon juice
1/4 teaspoon lemon peel, grated fine

1/2 teaspoon cinnamon
1 tablespoon arrowroot powder
Non-nutritive sweetener equivalent to 3/4 cup sugar

Pastry for one-crust pie

Preheat oven to 425°. Wash berries, mix with rest of ingredients. Put into unbaked pie crust and bake until tender (45-50 minutes). If a two-crust pie is desired, cover the pie before baking, cut vents in the top crust, flute edges, and cover fluting with foil to prevent excessive browning. *For a two-crust pie, adjust exchanges per serving to 2 bread, 3 fat, and add an additional 130 calories.*

**BANANA CREAM PIE

Exchanges per serving: 1 = 1/3 bread, 1/2 skim milk.

1 pastry = 1 bread, 1 1/2 fat.

Calories per serving: filling: 75

pastry: 135

Yield: 6 servings

1/4 cup flour
1 1/2 cups skim milk
1/4 cup (1 medium) egg
1 teaspoon lemon juice
1/2 teaspoon vanilla extract
Non-nutritive sweetener equivalent to 1/2 cup sugar

1/8 teaspoon salt
1 banana
Pastry for one-crust pie
Nondairy whipping cream (optional)

Blend flour with 1/2 cup cold skim milk. Scald remaining 1 cup skim milk and add flour-milk mixture and egg, lemon juice, vanilla extract, sweetener, and salt. Cook in top of double boiler, stirring until thick. Slice banana into baked, cooled pie shell. Spread cream filling over top; cool. Cover with nondairy whipping cream, if desired. Use immediately.

**OLGA'S PUMPKIN PIE

Exchanges per serving: 1 = 1 bread, 1/2 "B" vegetable.
Calories per serving: 100 (+ pudding mix)   Yield: 6 servings

1 1/2 cups cornflakes
1 teaspoon diet margarine, melted
1 tablespoon hot water
1/2 cup dietetic pancake and waffle topping

1 cup skim milk
2 envelopes dietetic butterscotch or vanilla pudding
1 cup pumpkin, canned or fresh cooked
1/4 cup (1 medium) egg

Preheat oven to 325°. Crush cornflakes. Mix margarine and water, add to cornflakes and mix thoroughly. Spread mixture evenly in a 9" pie pan; press firmly around edge with spatula. Bake 8-10 minutes. Cool. Blend rest of ingredients in saucepan; cook over medium heat, stirring constantly until mixture comes to a boil. Cool to room temperature; pour into previously prepared pie shell. Chill at least three hours before serving.

**MARTI'S APPLE CRISP

Exchanges per serving: 1 = 1 fat, 1 fruit, 1/2 bread, 1/2 meat.
Calories per serving: 155   Yield: 6 servings

4 apples, cored, peeled, and sliced
1/4 cup water
1/2 teaspoon fresh lemon juice
Non-nutritive sweetener equivalent to 2/3 cup sugar

1/2 cup flour
1/2 teaspoon cinnamon
1/2 teaspoon allspice
1/2 teaspoon salt
3 tablespoons diet margarine
1/2 cup Parmesan cheese, grated (optional)

Preheat oven to 325°. Grease a shallow baking dish and place apple slices on bottom. Combine water, lemon juice, and sweetener and pour over apples. Combine dry ingredients; cut in margarine until it is the consistency of large peas. Sprinkle over apples. If desired, cover with grated cheese.

**DEEP DISH APPLE PIE

Exchanges per serving: 1 = 1 bread, 1 1/2 fat, 1 fruit.
Calories per serving: 165   Yield: 8 servings

4 apples, pared and sliced fine
2 teaspoons lemon juice
1/2 teaspoon lemon rind, grated
1 1/8 teaspoons salt
1/4 teaspoon nutmeg
1/2 teaspoon cinnamon

Non-nutritive sweetener equivalent to 1 cup sugar
1/2 tablespoon arrowroot powder
1 cup flour, sifted
1/3 cup diet margarine
1/3 cup water

Preheat oven to 425°. Combine apples, lemon juice, lemon rind, nutmeg, cinnamon, sweetener, arrowroot and 1/8 teaspoon salt. Place in well-buttered 9" deep-dish pie plate. Combine flour and 1 teaspoon salt; cut in margarine until consistency of cornmeal. Blend in water; roll out as for a pie crust; place this on top of filling. Bake until crust is brown (about 35 minutes).

**FRUIT COBBLER

Exchanges per serving: 1 = 1 bread, 1 1/2 fruit, 1/4 meat.
Calories per serving: 150   Yield: 4 servings

2 cups water-packed fruit (cherries, etc.), unsweetened
1/4 teaspoon lemon juice
1/8 teaspoon almond extract
1/2 teaspoon arrowroot powder
2/3 cup juice from fruit
1/2 cup flour, sifted
1/8 teaspoon salt
3/4 teaspoon baking powder
1 tablespoon diet margarine
1/4 cup (1 medium) egg
2 tablespoons skim milk
Non-nutritive sweetener equivalent to 1/4 cup sugar

Preheat oven to 425°. Using shallow cake pan, make a layer of drained fruit. Combine lemon juice, almond extract, arrowroot powder, and drained fruit juice. Pour over fruit. Mix flour, salt, and baking powder, cutting in margarine until mixture is like coarse sugar. Mix egg, skim milk, and sweetener. Stir into dry ingredients and spoon onto fruit. Bake until browned (25-30 minutes). Serve warm.

**FRUIT FILLING FOR PIE

Exchanges per serving: 1 = 1 fruit.
                       1 crust = 1 bread, 1 1/2 fat.
Calories per serving: filling: 40   Yield: 8 servings
                      crust: 135

4 cups any fruit (apples, blueberries, fresh peaches, pears, orange sections, pineapple, seedless grapes, etc.)
Non-nutritive sweetener equivalent to 3/4 cup sugar
1 tablespoon arrowroot powder
1/4 teaspoon lemon peel, grated fine
2 teaspoons lemon juice
1/4 teaspoon nutmeg
1/2 teaspoon cinnamon
Pastry for one-crust pie

Preheat oven to 425°. Mix all ingredients together and place in uncooked pie crust. Bake until fruit is tender (about 45-50 minutes). If a two-crust pie is desired, cover unbaked pie with second crust, cut air vents in top, and flute edges. Cover fluted edges with foil to prevent excessive browning (remove foil after half an hour) and bake as before. *For a two-crust pie, adjust exchanges per serving to 2 bread, 3 fat, and add an additional 130 calories.*

**PEACHY PIE

Exchanges per serving: 1 = 1/2 bread, 2 fruit.
Calories per serving: 113

Yield: 6 servings

1 1/2 cups cornflakes
1 tablespoon diet margarine, melted
1 teaspoon hot water
4 cups unsweetened or fresh peaches, sliced
2 envelopes dietetic cherry gelatin

3 teaspoons lemon juice
1 teaspoon lemon rind, grated
1/4 cup nonfat dry milk solids
1/4 cup cold water
Non-nutritive sweetener equivalent to 3 tablespoons sugar

Preheat oven to 325°. Crush cornflakes. Mix margarine and hot water; add to cornflakes and mix thoroughly. Spread mixture evenly in 8" pie pan; press firmly around edge with spatula. Bake 8-10 minutes. Cool. Drain peaches, keeping the juice to dissolve the gelatin in, adding water to make 1 cup liquid. Heat almost to boiling. Add 2 tablespoons lemon juice and rind. Cool. Chop and add the peaches and chill until mixture begins to thicken. Mix nonfat dry milk solids, cold water, and rest of lemon juice; whip until mixture stands in peaks. Add sweetener and beat until mixture stands in very stiff peaks; very carefully fold gelatin-peach mixture into whipped milk; mix. Pour gently into pie shell above and serve chilled.

***YUMMY FRUIT TARTS

Exchanges per serving: 1 = 1 fat, 1/2 meat, 1 fruit.
1 pastry = 1 fat, 1/2 bread.
Calories per serving: filling: 145
pastry: 115

Yield: 6 tarts

1 tablespoon arrowroot powder
1/8 teaspoon salt
Non-nutritive sweetener equivalent to 1 cup sugar
1 cup fresh orange juice
1 cup unsweetened pineapple chunks

1/2 cup (2 medium) eggs, beaten
1 banana, sliced thin
1/4 cup dried coconut, shredded
1 recipe Lorene's Graham Cracker Crust

Combine arrowroot, salt, sweetener, and orange juice. Drain pineapple and set fruit aside, using liquid and sufficient water to make 1 cup. Combine liquid, arrowroot mixture, and beaten eggs. Cook over medium heat, stirring constantly, until mixture boils and thickens. Remove from heat. Chill, then fold in pineapple chunks, sliced banana, and coconut. Place into crust and chill until ready to serve.

***APPLE TORTE

Exchanges per serving: 1 = 1 bread, 3 fat, 1 1/4 fruit.
Calories per serving: 245   Yield: 12 servings

2 cups flour	3 tablespoons lemon juice
Non-nutritive sweetener equivalent to 1 1/3 cups sugar	1 cup water
	10 apples, peeled, cored, and sliced
3/4 cup diet margarine	1/2 cup white raisins
1/4 cup (1 medium) egg	1 teaspoon cinnamon

Preheat oven to 375°. Mix flour with 2/3 sweetener; crumble margarine into flour mixture with fingers until size of peas. Stir in egg with fork until well blended; work dough with hands until a smooth ball; divide into 3 sections. Wrap 1/3 dough in waxed paper and store in refrigerator until ready for top crust. Grease a 10" spring pan lightly and press remaining 2/3 of dough firmly and evenly over bottom and about 3/4 way up sides of pan. Set aside. Mix lemon juice and water; add apples a few at a time to the lemon-water to moisten each slice thoroughly. When apples are moistened, squeeze moisture out with hands and place apples in large bowl. Add raisins, balance of sweetener, and cinnamon. Stir and mix with apples. Place into crust. Roll refrigerated 1/3 dough on board which has been well floured, to 1" larger than pan. Fit dough over apples, pressing side and top together with wet fingers (so surface is flush with top). Prick pastry with fork several times. Bake 1 hour and 10 minutes. Cool 10 minutes; loosen but leave in pan until room temperature.

***PUMPKIN PIE

Exchanges per serving: 1 = 1/4 meat, 3/4 milk, 1/3 "B" vegetable.
Calories per serving: filling: 156   Yield: 8 servings
                       pastry: 135

1 1/2 cups canned or fresh cooked pumpkin	1/4-1/2 teaspoon nutmeg
	1/4-1/2 teaspoon cloves
Non-nutritive sweetener equivalent to 3/4 cup sugar	1/2 cup (2 medium) eggs, slightly beaten
1/2 teaspoon salt	1 1/4 cups milk
1 1/4 teaspoons cinnamon	2 cups evaporated milk
1/2-1 teaspoon ginger	One 9" unbaked pastry shell

Preheat oven to 400°. Combine pumpkin, sweetener, salt, and spices thoroughly; blend in eggs, milk, and evaporated milk. Pour into unbaked pastry shell. Bake until knife inserted between center and outside comes out clean. Serve cool.

***POLLY'S PUMPKIN PIE

Exchanges per serving: 1 = 1/4 meat, 1/2 milk, 1 "B" vegetable.
1 pastry = 1 bread, 1 1/2 fat.
Calories per serving: filling: 135   Yield: 8 servings
pastry: 135

Non-nutritive sweetener
equivalent to 1 cup sugar
1 1/2 teaspoons cinnamon
1/2 teaspoon allspice
1/2 teaspoon ginger
1/2 teaspoon nutmeg

1/2 teaspoon cloves
1 3/4 cups evaporated milk,
undiluted
1/2 cup (2 medium) eggs, well
beaten
1 1/2 cups canned pumpkin
Pastry for one 9" pie shell

Preheat oven to 425°. Combine sweetener and spices, stir in evaporated milk and eggs and add pumpkin. Beat until smooth. Pour mixture into a chilled 9" pie shell (do not prick bottom of shell). Bake at 425° for 15 minutes, then reduce heat to 350° and bake until silver knife inserted at center of pie comes out clean (about 35-40 minutes). Cool.

***CHIFFON PUMPKIN PIE

Exchanges per serving: 1 = 1/2 meat, 1/4 milk, 1 "B" vegetable.
1 pastry = 1 bread, 1 1/2 fat.
Calories per serving: filling: 85   Yield: 8 servings
pastry: 135

1 envelope unflavored gelatin
1 cup evaporated milk, undiluted
1/2 cup water
1 cup (4 medium) eggs, separated
1/2 teaspoon nutmeg
1/2 teaspoon cinnamon

1/4 teaspoon ginger
1/2 teaspoon salt
Non-nutritive sweetener
equivalent to 3/4 cup sugar
1 1/4 cups canned pumpkin,
mashed
Pastry for one 9" pie crust

Line a 9" pie plate with desired crust. Bake and cool. Combine first eight ingredients, reserving whites of eggs. Beat well. Stir and cook in top of double boiler until consistency of medium white sauce (about 10 minutes). Stir in sweetener. Place in refrigerator until cold. Beat whites until they form soft peaks. Fold pumpkin into gelatin mixture; add beaten egg whites carefully. Pour into pie shell and chill until set.

***CHIFFON EGGNOG PIE

Exchanges per serving: 1 = 1/2 fat, 1/4 skim milk.
                     1 pastry = 1 bread, 1 1/2 fat.
Calories per serving: filling: 70   Yield: 6 servings
                     pastry: 135

1 envelope unflavored gelatin
1/4 cup cold water
1 1/2 cups skim milk
Non-nutritive sweetener
  equivalent to 3/4 cup sugar
1/4 teaspoon salt

1/2 tablespoon arrowroot
  powder
1/4 cup (1 medium) egg, separated
1 teaspoon almond extract
1 tablespoon rum extract

Pastry for one 9" pie shell

Soften gelatin in cold water. Combine 1/2 of the skim milk, sweetener, and salt in top of double boiler. Make a paste from arrowroot powder and remaining milk; stir into first mixture. Cook over boiling water. Stir constantly until thick; beat egg yolks and add a little of the hot mixture to them; stir this into remaining hot liquid in double boiler. Cook another 2 minutes; remove from heat and stir in softened gelatin until dissolved. Chill until mixture begins to set, then stir in extracts. Beat egg whites very stiff and fold into gelatin mixture. Pour into baked pie shell and chill until firm. If desired, top with Low-Calorie Topping Whip or artificial whipped cream and sprinkle chocolate shavings over this.

***JIFFY BANANA CREAM PIE

Exchanges per serving: 1/8 filling = 1 fruit, 1/2 skim milk.
                     1/8 pastry = 1 bread, 1 1/2 fat.
Calories per serving: filling: 80
                     pastry: 135   Yield: 1 pie
                     pudding mix: consult package

2 packages dietetic vanilla
  pudding mix
2 cups skim milk

2 bananas, sliced (or other
  fruit such as peaches, strawberries, etc.)

Prepare pudding mix using the skim milk; cool slightly. Line 8" pie pan with desired baked crust. Place banana slices to cover bottom of shell; fill with pudding and let stand until set.

***GREAT APPLE AND GRAPE PIE

Exchanges per serving: 1 = 1/2 fat, 2 fruit.

1 pastry = 1 bread, 1 1/2 fat.

Calories per serving: filling: 105   Yield: 6 servings

pastry: 135

3 tablespoons tapioca
1/16 teaspoon salt
3 cups apples, cored, pared, and sliced
2 cups seedless grapes, cut in halves
1/2 cup water

Non-nutritive sweetener equivalent to 1 cup sugar
2 tablespoons lemon juice
1 tablespoon diet margarine, melted
Pastry for one 9" pie shell, unbaked

Preheat oven to 425°. Mix tapioca and salt and toss with apples and grapes. Place into unbaked pie shell. Combine remaining ingredients and place over fruit. Cover top with aluminum foil and bake 15 minutes. Reduce heat to 325° and continue baking until apples are tender (about 50 minutes).

***MARY C'S PUMPKIN PIE

Exchanges per serving: 1 filling = 1/4 milk, 1 "B" vegetable.

1 pastry = 1 bread, 1 1/2 fat.

Calories per serving: filling: 100   Yield: 6 servings

pastry: 135

1/4 cup (1 medium) egg
Non-nutritive sweetener equivalent to 1 cup sugar
3/4 teaspoon allspice
3/4 teaspoon nutmeg
3/4 teaspoon cinnamon

1/2 teaspoon ginger
1/4 teaspoon cloves, finely grated
1 1/2 cups canned pumpkin
3/4 cup evaporated milk
3/4 cup fresh orange juice

One 9" pastry shell, unbaked

Preheat oven to 425°. Combine egg, sweetener, spices, and pumpkin and blend well. Add milk and orange juice gradually; stir until well blended. Pour into unbaked pie shell. Bake 10-12 minutes, then reduce heat to 325° and bake until a knife inserted near center comes out clean (about 3/4 hour).

****APPLE PIE

Exchanges per serving: 1 filling = 1 fruit, 1/2 fat.

1 pastry = 2 bread, 3 fat.

Calories per serving: filling: 75   Yield: 8 servings

pastry: 265

3 cups tart apples
Non-nutritive sweetener equivalent to 3/4 cup sugar
2 tablespoons flour

1/2 teaspoon cinnamon
1/16 teaspoon nutmeg
1/16 teaspoon salt
Pastry for two-crust 9" pie

2 tablespoons diet margarine

Preheat oven to 400°. Pare apples and slice thin. Combine sweetener, flour, spices, and salt; mix with apples. Line pie plate with pastry; fill with apple mixture and dot with margarine. Place top crust on pie and sprinkle with sugar substitute, if desired. Bake about 50 minutes, or until done.

****QUICK APPLE PIE

Exchanges per serving: 1 = 1 fruit.
1 pastry = 2 bread, 3 fat.
Calories per serving: filling: 40   Yield: 8 servings
pastry: 265

4 cups apples, pared, and sliced very thin
2 teaspoons lemon juice
1/4 teaspoon lemon peel, grated fine
1/4 teaspoon nutmeg
1/2 teaspoon cinnamon

1 tablespoon arrowroot powder
Non-nutritive sweetener equivalent to 3/4 cup sugar
Pastry for two-crust Flaky Pie Crust

Preheat oven to 425°. Mix together everything except the pastry. Prepare crust, lining an 8" pie plate. Fill with apple mix and top with second crust; flute edges. Make four or five cuts for air vents. Lightly cover fluted edges with aluminum foil to prevent excessive browning of crust. After about 30 minutes remove foil and continue baking until apples are tender (another 10-20 minutes). Cool.

****SHERRY'S APPLE PIE

Exchanges per serving: 1 = 1 fruit.
1 pastry = 2 bread, 3 fat.
Calories per serving: filling: 40   Yield: 6 servings
pastry: 265

5 apples, sliced
2 teaspoons tapioca
Non-nutritive sweetener equivalent to 1/2 cup sugar

1/16 teaspoon cinnamon
Pastry for one-crust pie

Preheat oven to 400°. Roll 1/2 of the crust recipe to fit a 9" pie pan; arrange apple slices in crust; sprinkle tapioca, sweetener, and cinnamon over top. Roll out remaining crust and crimp edges securely over top (moisten edges between crusts with water if necessary), and perforate in about half dozen places. Bake until apples are tender (about 30 minutes). *If a one-crust pie is desired adjust exchange per serving to 1 bread, 1 1/2 fat, and subtract 130 calories per serving.*

*RICE CEREAL PIE CRUST

Exchanges per serving: 1 serving = 1 fat.
Calories per serving: 50   Yield: 8 servings

1 cup crispy rice cereal, crushed
2 tablespoons diet margarine, melted

Non-nutritive sweetener equivalent to 4 tablespoons sugar

Mix ingredients together and line bottom and sides of 8" pan. Chill well before adding any desired filling.

*CRUMBLY PIE CRUST

Exchanges per serving: 1" slice = 1/2 fat.
Calories per serving: 35   Yield: One 10" crust

3 tablespoons diet margarine
Non-nutritive sweetener equivalent to 1 tablespoon sugar

3/4 cup cornflake crumbs

Preheat oven to 375°. Mix margarine, sweetener, and crumbs; press into 9" pie plate, with back of spoon. Press into bottom and up sides of plate (crust will be fairly thin).

**RICH FLAKY CRUST

Exchanges per serving: 1 = 1 bread, 1 1/2 fat.
Calories per serving: 135   Yield: Two 8" crusts

2 cups flour, sifted
1 teaspoon salt

1/2 cup oil
3 tablespoons cold water

Preheat oven to 450°. Sift flour and salt together, then dribble oil on surface. Stir with fork until completely mixed. Add cold water to form smooth ball. Divide dough in half. Place on waxed paper, cover with another piece of waxed paper, roll dough to 12" circle. Peel off paper and fit into pie plate; flute edges with fork (or finger) which has been moistened. Bake until browned (12-15 minutes). Cool before filling. For two-crust pie, place one crust (unbaked) into pie plate, put in filling and top with other crust which has been slit in several places. Bake according to filling instructions. *For two-crust pie, allow 2 bread and 3 fat exchanges, and adjust calories to 265 per serving.*

**PIE CRUST

Exchanges per serving: 1 = 1 1/4 bread, 2 fat.
Calories per serving: 190
Yield: 8 servings

1 1/3 cups flour, sifted
1/2 teaspoon salt

1/2 cup diet margarine, melted

2 tablespoons cold water

Sift flour and salt together, then dribble margarine over surface. Stir
with fork until completely mixed. Add water over margarine and flour
mixture and stir to smooth ball. Roll out dough to fit 8" pie plate. Flute
edges with fork. Refrigerate if crust is to be filled prior to baking. If
baked unfilled, make several cuts with sharp knife in bottom and sides
of crust. Bake at 450° until golden brown (13-15 minutes).

**LORENE'S GRAHAM CRACKER CRUST

Exchanges per serving: 1 = 1 bread, 1 fat.
Calories per serving: 115
Yield: 9 servings

1 cup graham crackers,
crushed fine
3 tablespoons diet margarine,
melted

Non-nutritive sweetener
equivalent to 2 tablespoons
sugar

Preheat oven to 350°. Combine ingredients well and press firmly into a
9" pie plate. Bake about 10 minutes. Chill before filling.

**PASTRY

Exchanges per serving: 1/8 crust = 1 bread, 1 1/2 fat.
Calories per serving: 135
Yield: One 8" crust

1 cup flour, sifted
1 teaspoon salt

5 tablespoons diet margarine
4 tablespoons water

Preheat oven to 425°. Combine flour and salt. Cut in margarine until
consistency of peas. Add water slowly until the dough is moistened and
holds together. Roll dough, pressing into a ball. Flour pastry board and
rolling pin and roll gently, turning often. Roll thin, lay pastry over 8"
pie tin and press down gently, fluting edges. Slit bottom a few times
with a sharp knife. Bake until golden brown (about 14-15 minutes). Fill
with desired filling. Use extra dough for individual pastries.

CANNING AND FREEZING
and
JAMS AND JELLIES

CANNING FRUITS

To can fruits, use unsweetened fruit juice or water in place of the usual sugar-syrup. Be sure to adhere to processing time and other instructions, and when serving, count your fruit exchanges as you would for the commercially prepared sugar-free fruits.

Soak the fruit in lemon juice solution to keep it from darkening. Use sweetener equivalent to 2-4 cups of sugar for every 2-3 quarts of liquid; if this is not sweet enough (or yet too sweet) change it to suit your taste. The U. S. Department of Agriculture, Washington, D. C., 20402, has some excellent books on canning which you may wish to send for before trying any recipes. They cost about 20 cents each.

Use orange or pineapple juice, unsweetened, to obtain an unusual flavor. (These generally settle to the bottom of the jars, so shake well just before serving.) Another good variation is a half-and-half mixture of peaches and pears.

Raspberries and strawberries may be mashed and the juice saved; mixing this juice with water makes an excellent canning liquid.

Apples, grapes, peaches, pears, pineapple, and seedless oranges are fine to mix. Avoid fruits such as bananas, blueberries, cherries, plums, raspberries, and strawberries in fruit cocktail. (Bananas turn brown and become too soft, while the other fruits "weep" and become too liquid.)

Plums are fine for canning, but be sure you select the proper varieties. Use half water and half plum juice for the canning liquid to help keep the color from being lost.

FREEZING FRUITS WITHOUT SUGAR

Wash and drain thoroughly blackberries, blueberries, cranberries, currants, gooseberries, grapes, pineapple chunks, plums, raspberries, or rhubarb. Leave about 1/2 inch at top of container when packing. Freeze.

Figs, peaches, and strawberries go into special containers, covered with the ascorbic acid water solution (1 teaspoon ascorbic acid — crystalline — to each quart of water). Package, leaving 1 inch at top of quarts and 1/2 inch for pints. Freeze. Thaw frozen fruits until all but a few ice crystals remain and sweeten as desired with non-nutritive sweetener.

JAMS AND JELLIES WITHOUT SUGAR

Cover jars completely with water and bring water to boil. Boil 15-20 minutes. Then remove jars from water (hold tongs under boiling water 60-90 seconds before removing jars so jars do not break); drain jars upside down on aluminum foil paper until just before using, then turn to right side up.

Use your favorite non-nutritive sweetener, being careful to use proper amount needed. Stir until it is completely dissolved and mixed. (Do not reboil.)

In top of double boiler, over low heat, melt the paraffin. Pour jam or jellies into jars carefully, and pour on melted paraffin about 1/4 inch thickness. Cool. Place in refrigerator. Keep refrigerated, and after first opening, be sure to keep covered with tight lid or aluminum foil molded to top.

VEGETABLES

Nearly any vegetable which can be cooked is recommended for freezing. Order the freezing booklet from the Department of Agriculture, Washington, D. C. 20402 (15-20¢).

*CUCUMBER PICKLES

Exchanges per serving: 1 pint = None.
Calories per serving: 0

Yield: 3 pints

6 cucumbers
1/4 cup salt
Non-nutritive sweetener equivalent to 3/4 cup sugar

1/4 cup water
2 cups white vinegar
2 tablespoons pickling spice

Wash and dry cucumbers, cut into strips about 4" long. Place in large bowl and sprinkle with salt. Let stand overnight. In the morning rinse and drain well several times. Combine sweetener, water, and vinegar in large pan and bring to boil. Tie pickling spice in a cheesecloth bag and add to boiling ingredients. Add cucumbers and reduce heat; simmer about 15 minutes. Place cucumbers in clean hot pint jars. Heat liquid once more to boiling point, and pour over pickles in jars. Seal immediately.

*APPLE BUTTER JELLY

Exchanges per serving: 1 tablespoon = 1/4 fruit.
Calories per serving: 10

Serves 5 3/4 cups

8 cups apples, washed and cut in quarters
2 cups unsweetened apple juice
1/4 cup lemon juice
1/4 cup cider vinegar
2 teaspoons lemon peel, ground fine

1/4 teaspoon nutmeg
1 teaspoon cloves
1/4 teaspoon anise seed, ground fine
Non-nutritive sweetener equivalent to 1/2 cup sugar

Prepare jelly jars. Mix all ingredients except sweetener. Bring to a boil, stirring constantly; boil a few minutes. Remove from heat, then stir in sweetener. Seal jars.

*ANNE'S CHILI SAUCE

Exchanges per serving: 1 tablespoon = 1 "A" vegetable.
Calories per serving: 6   Yield: 3 quarts

8 cups tomatoes, peeled and chopped
1/4 cup red peppers, chopped fine
1/2 cup green peppers, chopped fine
1 1/2 cups onion, chopped fine
1 1/2 cups celery, chopped fine

Non-nutritive sweetener equivalent to 1/2 cup sugar
1 tablespoon salt
1 1/2 cups cider vinegar
1 tablespoon Tabasco sauce
1 whole stick cinnamon
1 teaspoon cloves
1 1/2 teaspoons celery seed
1 1/2 teaspoons mustard seed
1 teaspoon Mei Yen seasoning

In a large heavy pan combine first nine ingredients. Combine spices in a cheesecloth bag and add to first mixture. Bring to boil; reduce heat and simmer. Stir occasionally, simmering for about 5-6 hours. Remove bag of spices, pour remainder into clean, hot, pint jars and seal immediately.

*RUTH'S RASPBERRY JAM

Exchanges per serving: 1 tablespoon = 1/8 fruit.
Calories per serving: 5   Yield: 2 cups

1 1/2 teaspoons unflavored gelatin
1 1/2 tablespoons cold water
3 cups fresh raspberries, crushed

Non-nutritive sweetener equivalent to 2/3 cup sugar
1/4 teaspoon lemon juice
3 drops red food coloring (optional)

Soften gelatin in cold water. Combine berries and sweetener in saucepan; place on high heat. Stir constantly until mixture boils, then remove from heat and add softened gelatin. Return to heat and cook for another minute. Remove and blend in lemon juice and food coloring. Place in pint jar. Seal and store in refrigerator.

*ANNE'S APPLE JELLY

Exchanges per serving: 1 tablespoon = 1/4 fruit.
Calories per serving: 10   Yield: 2 cups

2 teaspoons unflavored gelatin
2 tablespoons lemon juice
1/8 teaspoon salt
1 teaspoon arrowroot powder

2 cups apple juice, unsweetened
Non-nutritive sweetener equivalent to 2 cups sugar

Prepare jelly jars. Mix the gelatin, lemon juice, salt, and arrowroot. Then stir in apple juice and boil, stirring constantly, for two minutes. Remove from heat. Stir in sweetener. Fill jelly jars, seal, and store.

*BLUEBERRY JAM

Exchanges per serving: 1 tablespoon = 1/4 fruit.
Calories per serving: 10 Yield: 2 1/2 cups

2 tablespoons lemon juice
3 teaspoons unflavored gelatin
1/8 teaspoon salt
1 1/2 teaspoons arrowroot powder

2 1/2 cups frozen unsweetened blueberries, partially thawed
Non-nutritive sweetener equivalent to 2 cups sugar

Prepare jelly jars. Mix lemon juice, gelatin, salt, and arrowroot, then stir in blueberries. Boil gently until mixture thickens, stirring constantly (about 3-4 minutes). Stir constantly, boiling at full boil for 2 minutes. Remove from heat; stir in sweetener. Fill jars.

*PHYL'S APPLE JELLY

Exchanges per serving: 1 tablespoon = 1/4 fruit.
Calories per serving: 10 Yield: 2 cups

4 teaspoons unflavored gelatin
2 cups unsweetened apple juice
Non-nutritive sweetener equivalent to 1 cup sugar

1 1/2 teaspoons lemon juice
3 drops food coloring (yellow or green)

Soften gelatin in 1/4 of the apple juice; bring rest of juice to boil. Remove from heat; add softened gelatin. Stir until dissolved; add sweetener, lemon juice, and food coloring. Bring to rolling boil. Place in clean pint jars; seal. Store in refrigerator.

*APPLE-LEMON JELLY

Exchanges per serving: 1/2 cup = 1 fruit.
Calories per serving: 40 Yield: 2 cups

1 package unflavored gelatin
2 tablespoons lemon juice
1/8 teaspoon salt
1 teaspoon arrowroot powder

2 cups apple juice, unsweetened
Non-nutritive sweetener equivalent to 2 cups sugar

Mix gelatin, lemon juice, salt, and arrowroot powder. Add apple juice and boil, stirring constantly, for two minutes. Remove from heat; add sweetener. Fill prepared jelly jars; seal.

*STRAWBERRY JELLY

Exchanges per serving: 1 tablespoon = 1/4 fruit.
Calories per serving: 10   Yield: 5 1/2 cups

2 envelopes unflavored gelatin
1/2 cup lemon juice
1/16 teaspoon salt
1 tablespoon arrowroot powder

4 cups strawberries, hulled, washed, and strained
Non-nutritive sweetener equivalent to 4 cups sugar

Mix gelatin, lemon juice, salt, and arrowroot, then add strawberries. Boil, stirring constantly, about 3 minutes. Remove from heat; stir in sweetener. Fill jars. Seal.

*PINEAPPLE-APRICOT JAM

Exchanges per serving: 1 tablespoon = 1/2 fruit.
Calories per serving: 20   Yield: 5 cups

2 cups dried apricots
2 cups water
4 cups unsweetened pineapple tidbits

2 tablespoons lemon juice
1/16 teaspoon salt
Non-nutritive sweetener equivalent to 1 cup sugar

Boil apricots in water until tender (about 25 minutes). Drain pineapple tidbits and cut each one in half. Puree apricots and water with lemon juice and salt. Return to saucepan and stir in pineapple. Boil a few minutes, stirring now and then. Remove from heat; add sweetener. Fill jelly jars, seal.

*CONSERVE

Exchanges per serving: 1 tablespoon = 1/2 fat, 1/2 fruit.
Calories per serving: 42   Yield: 2 cups

1 cup dried apricots
2 cups water
2 1/4 cups unsweetened pineapple tidbits

1/8 teaspoon salt
2 tablespoons lemon juice
Non-nutritive sweetener equivalent to 1 cup sugar

1/2 cup nuts, finely chopped

Boil apricots in water until tender. Puree. Drain pineapple tidbits, cut each piece into smaller pieces. Blend puree of apricots and water in saucepan; add pineapple, then salt and lemon juice. Boil slowly, stirring constantly, about 5 minutes. Remove from heat and stir in sweetener and nuts. Fill jars.

*JOAN'S CHUTNEY

Exchanges per serving: 1/4 cup = 1 1/2 fruit.
Calories per serving: 60   Yield: 1 1/2 pints

3/4 cup white raisins
1/4 cup bell peppers, chopped fine
1 cup white vinegar
4 pears, cored, pared, and chopped

Non-nutritive sweetener equivalent to 2 cups sugar
1/2 teaspoon ginger
1/4 teaspoon allspice
1/4 teaspoon cloves
1/4 teaspoon salt

Combine all the ingredients in large pan and bring to boil. Reduce heat to medium and cook until pears are tender and mixture is slightly thick (about an hour). Spoon into clean jars and seal immediately.

TABLES AND CHARTS

HEIGHT AND WEIGHT CHARTS

DESIRABLE WEIGHT CHART FOR WOMEN, DRESSED
(but minus coats, hats, purse, etc.)

Height (with shoes)	Small Frame	Medium Frame	Large Frame	Calorie Intake
4 ft. 10 in.	92-98	96-107	104-119	1200-1500
4 ft. 11 in.	94-101	98-110	106-122	1200-1500
5 ft. 0 in.	96-104	98-110	109-125	1200-1500
5 ft. 1 in.	99-107	104-116	112-128	1250-1575
5 ft. 2 in.	102-110	107-119	115-131	1300-1650
5 ft. 3 in.	105-113	110-122	118-134	1350-1725
5 ft. 4 in.	108-116	113-126	121-138	1450-1800
5 ft. 5 in.	111-119	116-130	125-142	1500-1850
5 ft. 6 in.	114-123	120-135	129-146	1550-1950
5 ft. 7 in.	118-127	124-139	133-150	1600-2000
5 ft. 8 in.	122-131	128-143	137-154	1650-2100
5 ft. 9 in.	126-135	132-147	141-158	1750-2200
5 ft. 10 in.	130-140	136-151	145-163	1800-2300
5 ft. 11 in.	134-144	140-155	149-168	1850-2300
6 ft. 0 in.	138-148	144-159	153-173	1900-2400

DESIRABLE WEIGHT CHART FOR MEN, DRESSED
(without outer garments, coat, hats., etc.)

Height (with shoes)	Small Frame	Medium Frame	Large Frame	Calorie Intake
5 ft. 2 in.	112-120	118-129	126-141	1500-1850
5 ft. 3 in.	115-123	121-133	129-144	1500-1900
5 ft. 4 in.	118-126	124-136	132-148	1550-1950
5 ft. 5 in.	121-129	127-139	135-152	1650-2050
5 ft. 6 in.	124-133	130-143	138-156	1700-2150
5 ft. 7 in.	128-137	134-147	142-161	1750-2200
5 ft. 8 in.	132-141	138-152	147-166	1850-2300
5 ft. 9 in.	136-145	142-156	151-170	1900-2400
5 ft. 10 in.	140-150	146-160	155-174	1950-2500
5 ft. 11 in.	144-154	150-165	159-179	2050-2550
6 ft. 0 in.	148-158	154-170	164-184	2100 2650
6 ft. 1 in.	152-162	158-175	168-189	2150-2800
6 ft. 2 in.	156-167	162-180	173-194	2250-2850
6 ft. 3 in.	160-171	167-185	178-199	2300-2900
6 ft. 4 in.	164-175	172-190	182-204	2400-3000

Courtesy Eli Lilly and Company, Indianapolis, Indiana

NUTRITIVE VALUES OF THE EDIBLE PART OF FOOD

Food, approximate measure, and weight (in grams)		Carbo-hy-drate	Fat (total lipid)	Fatty Acids			Food Energy	Pro-tein	Water
				Satu-rated (total)	Unsaturated Oleic	Linoleic			
	grams	grams	grams	grams	grams	grams	Calories	grams	Percent
FATS, OILS									
Butter, 4 sticks per pound:									
Sticks, 2 ....1 cup	227	45	184	101	61	6	1,625	1	16
Stick, 1/8 ....1 tablespoon	14	3	11	6	4	trace	100	trace	16
Pat or square (64 per lb.) 1 pat..............	7	1	6	3	2	trace	50	trace	16
Fats, cooking:									
Lard ....1 cup	200	0	220	84	101	22	1,985	0	0
Lard ....1 tablespoon	14	0	14	5	6	1	125	0	0
Vegetable fats ......1 cup	200	0	200	46	130	14	1,770	0	0
Vegetable fats ......1 tablespoon	12.5	0	12	3	8	1	110	0	0
Margarine, 4 sticks per pound:									
Sticks, 2 ....1 cup	227	1	184	37	105	33	1,635	1	16
Stick, 1/8 ....1 tablespoon	14	trace	11	2	6	2	100	trace	16
Pat or square (64 per pound) 1 pat..............	7	trace	6	1	3	1	50	trace	16
Oils, salad or cooking:									
Corn...............1 tablespoon	14	0	14	1	4	7	125	0	0
Cottonseed ....1 tablespoon	14	0	14	4	3	7	125	0	0
Olive..............1 tablespoon	14	0	14	2	11	1	125	0	0
Soybean............1 tablespoon	14	0	14	2	3	7	125	0	0
Salad dressings:									
Blue cheese.........1 tablespoon	16	1	8	2	2	4	80	1	32
Commercial, mayonnaise type.........1 tablespoon	15	2	6	1	1	3	65	trace	41

NUTRITIVE VALUES OF THE EDIBLE PART OF FOOD

Food, approximate measure, and weight (in grams)		Carbohydrate	Fat (total lipid)	Fatty Acids			Food Energy	Protein	Water
				Saturated (total)	Unsaturated				
					Oleic	Linoleic			
	grams	grams	grams	grams	grams	grams	Calories	grams	Percent
French ....1 tablespoon.....	15	3	6	1	1	3	60	trace	39
Home cooked, boiled.........1 tablespoon.....	17	3	2	1	1	trace	30	1	68
Mayonnaise..........1 tablespoon.....	15	trace	12	2	3	6	110	trace	15
Thousand Island .....1 tablespoon.....	15	2	8	1	2	4	75	trace	32
FRUITS AND FRUIT PRODUCTS									
Apples, raw, medium 2 1/2 inch. dia., about 3 per lb¹.....1 apple	150	18	trace				70	trace	85
Apple Brown Betty ..1 cup	230	68	8	4	3	trace	345	4	64
Apple Juice, bottled or canned.1 cup	249	30	trace				120	trace	88
Applesauce canned:									
Sweetened ....1 cup	254	60	trace				230	1	76
Unsweetened or artificially sweetened...........1 cup	239	26	trace				100	trace	88
Applesauce and apricots, canned, strained or junior (baby food) ..1 ounce	28	6	trace				25	trace	77
Apricots: Raw, about 12 per pound¹............3 apricots	114	14	trace				55	1	85

¹-Measure and weight apply to entire vegetable or fruit including parts not usually eaten.

NUTRITIVE VALUES OF THE EDIBLE PART OF FOOD

Food, approximate measure, and weight (in grams)		Carbohydrate	Fat (total lipid)	Fatty Acids			Food Energy	Protein	Water
				Saturated (total)	Unsaturated Oleic	Linoleic			
	grams	grams	grams	grams	grams	grams	Calories	grams	Percent
Canned in heavy syrup:									
Halves and syrup...1 cup	259	57	trace				220	2	77
Halves (medium) and syrup......4 halves; 2 tablespoons	122	27	trace				105	1	77
Dried:									
Uncooked, 40 halves, small......1 cup	150	100	1				390	8	25
Cooked, unsweetened, fruit and liquid......1 cup	285	62	1				240	5	76
Apricot nectar, canned......1 cup	250	36	trace				140	1	85
Avocado, raw: California varieties, mainly Fuerte: 10-ounce avocado, about 3 1/2 inches by 4 1/4 inches, peeled and pitted......1/2 avocado	108	6	18	4	8	2	185	2	74
1/2-inch cubes......1 cup	152	9	26	5	12	3	260	3	74

[1]·Measure and weight apply to entire vegetable or fruit including parts not usually eaten.

NUTRITIVE VALUES OF THE EDIBLE PART OF FOOD

Food, approximate measure, and weight (in grams)	Carbohydrate	Fat (total lipid)	Fatty Acids Saturated (total)	Unsaturated Oleic	Linoleic	Food Energy	Protein	Water
grams	grams	grams	grams	grams	grams	Calories	grams	Percent
Florida varieties: 13-ounce avocado, about 4 inches by 3 inches, peeled and pitted .... 1/2 avocado 123	11	14	3	6	2	160	2	78
1/2-inch cubes ....1 cup 152	13	17	3	8	2	195	2	78
Bananas, raw, 6 by 1 1/2 inches, about 3 per pound[1] ....1 banana.......... 150	23	trace				85	1	76
Blackberries, raw .....1 cup 144	19	1				85	2	84
Blueberries, raw .....1 cup 140	21	1				85	1	83
Cantaloupes, raw; medium, 5-inch dia., about 1 2/3 pounds[1] ....1/2 melon 385	14	trace				60	1	91
Cherries: Raw, sweet, with stems[1].............1 cup 130	20	trace				80	2	80
Canned, red, sour, pitted, heavy syrup ....1 cup 260	59	1				230	2	76
Cranberry juice cocktail, canned .....1 cup 250	41	trace				160	trace	83
Cranberry sauce, sweetened, canned, strained ....1 cup 277	104	1				405	trace	62

[1]-Measure and weight apply to entire vegetable or fruit including parts not usually eaten.

NUTRITIVE VALUES OF THE EDIBLE PART OF FOOD

Food, approximate measure, and weight (in grams)		Carbo-hy-drate	Fat (total lipid)	Fatty Acids			Food Energy	Pro-tein	Water
				Satu-rated (total)	Unsaturated Oleic	Lino-leic			
	grams	grams	grams	grams	grams	grams	Calo-ries	grams	Per-cent
Dates, domestic, natural and dry, pitted, cut ....1 cup	178	130	1				490	4	22
Figs: Raw, small 1 1/2 inch dia., about 12 per pound ....3 figs	114	23	trace				90	1	78
Dried, large, 2 inch by 1 inch ..1 fig	21	15	trace				60	1	23
Fruit cocktail: canned in heavy syrup, solids and liquid ....1 cup	256	50	1				195	1	80
Grapefruit: Raw, medium, 4 1/4 inch diameter, size 64: White[1] ......1/2 grapefruit	285	14	trace				55	1	89
Pink or red[1] ......1/2 grapefruit	285	15	trace				60	1	89
Raw sections, white ....1 cup	194	20	trace				75	1	89
Canned, white: Syrup pack, solids and liquid ....1 cup	249	44	trace				175	1	81

[1]-Measure and weight apply to entire vegetable or fruit including parts not usually eaten.

NUTRITIVE VALUES OF THE EDIBLE PART OF FOOD

Food, approximate measure, and weight (in grams)	grams	Carbo-hy-drate grams	Fat (total lipid) grams	Fatty Acids Satu-rated (total) grams	Oleic grams	Lino-leic grams	Food Energy Calo-ries	Pro-tein grams	Water Per-cent
Water pack, solids and liquid ....1 cup	240	18	trace				70	1	91
Grapefruit juice:									
Fresh ....1 cup	246	23	trace				95	1	90
Canned white:									
Unsweetened .....1 cup	247	24	trace				100	1	89
Sweetened ....1 cup	250	32	trace				130	1	86
Frozen, concentrate, unsweetened:									
Undiluted, can 6 fluid ounces ....1 can	207	72	1				300	4	62
Diluted with 3 parts water, by volume.......1 cup	247	24	trace				100	1	89
Frozen, concentrate, sweetened:									
Undiluted, can, 6 fluid ounces ....1 can	211	85	1				350	3	57
Diluted with 3 parts water, by volume ....1 cup	249	28	trace				115	1	88
Dehydrated:									
Crystals, can, net weight 4 ounces...1 can	114	103	1				430	5	1

NUTRITIVE VALUES OF THE EDIBLE PART OF FOOD

Food, approximate measure, and weight (in grams)	grams	Carbohydrate grams	Fat (total lipid) grams	Fatty Acids Saturated (total) grams	Unsaturated Oleic grams	Linoleic grams	Food Energy Calories	Protein grams	Water percent
Prepared with water (1 pound yields about 1 gallon)....1 cup	247	24	trace				100	1	90
Grapes, raw:									
American type (slip skin), such as Concord, Delaware, Niagara, Catawba, and Scuppernong[1].......1 cup	153	15	1				65	1	82
European type (adherent), such as Malaga, Muscat, Thompson Seedless, Emperor, and Flame Tokay....1 cup	160	25	trace				95	1	81
Grape juice, bottled or canned....1 cup	254	42	trace				165	1	83
Lemons, raw, medium, 2-1/5-inch diameter, size 150......1 lemon	106	6	trace				20	1	90
Lemon juice:									
Fresh......1 cup	246	20	trace				60	1	91
1 tablespoon	15	1	trace				5	trace	91
Canned, unsweetened......1 cup	245	19	trace				55	1	92
Lemonade concentrate, frozen, sweetened:									

[1]-Measure and weight apply to entire vegetable or fruit including parts not usually eaten.

NUTRITIVE VALUES OF THE EDIBLE PART OF FOOD

Food, approximate measure, and weight (in grams)		Carbohydrate	Fat (total lipid)	Fatty Acids Saturated (total)	Unsaturated Oleic	Linoleic	Food Energy	Protein	Water
	grams	grams	grams	grams	grams	grams	Calories	grams	Percent
Undiluted, can, 6 fluid ounces ..... 1 can	220	112	trace				430	trace	48
Diluted with 4 1/3 parts water, by volume .... 1 cup	248	28	trace				110	trace	88
Lime juice:									
Fresh .... 1 cup	246	22	trace				65	1	90
Canned.......... 1 cup	246	22	trace				65	1	90
Limeade concentrate, frozen, sweetened:									
Undiluted, can 6 fluid ounces ..... 1 can	218	108	trace				410	trace	50
Diluted with 4 1/3 parts water, by volume .... 1 cup	248	27	trace				105	trace	90
Oranges, raw:									
California, Navel (winter), 2-4/5-inch diameter, size 88[1] .... 1 orange	180	16	trace				60	2	85
Florida, all varieties, 3-inch diameter ...... 1 orange	210	19	trace				75	1	86
Orange juice: Fresh: California, Valencia (summer) .... 1 cup	249	26	1				115	2	88

[1]-Measure and weight apply to entire vegetable or fruit including parts not usually eaten.

NUTRITIVE VALUES OF THE EDIBLE PART OF FOOD

Food, approximate measure, and weight (in grams)	grams	Carbo-hydrate grams	Fat (total lipid) grams	Fatty Acids Saturated (total) grams	Unsaturated Oleic grams	Linoleic grams	Food Energy Calories	Protein grams	Water Percent
Florida varieties:									
Early and mid-season............1 cup............	247	23	trace				100	1	90
Late season, Valencia...........1 cup............	248	26	trace				110	1	88
Canned, unsweetened ....1 cup............	249	28	trace				120	2	87
Frozen concentrate:									
Undiluted, can, 6 fluid ounces ....1 can............	210	80	trace				330	5	58
Diluted with 3 parts water, by volume.1 cup............	248	27	trace				110	2	88
Dehydrated:									
Crystals, can, net weight 4 ounces...1 can............	113	100	2				430	6	1
Prepared with water, 1 pound yields about 1 gallon ....1 cup............	248	27	trace				115	1	88
Orange and grapefruit juice:									
Frozen concentrate:									
Undiluted, can, 6 fluid ounces......1 can....	209	78	1				325	4	59
Diluted with 3 parts water, by volume.1 cup............	248	26	trace				110	1	88
Papayas, raw, 1/2-inch cubes.................1 cup.............	182	18	trace				70	1	89

NUTRITIVE VALUES OF THE EDIBLE PART OF FOOD

Food, approximate measure, and weight (in grams)		Carbo-hy-drate	Fat (total lipid)	Fatty Acids			Food Energy	Pro-tein	Water
				Satu-rated (total)	Unsaturated				
					Oleic	Lino-leic			
	grams	grams	grams	grams	grams	grams	Calo-ries	grams	Per-cent
Peaches:									
Raw:									
Whole, medium, 2-inch diameter, about 4 per									
pound..........1 peach..........	114	10	trace				35	1	89
Sliced............1 cup	168	16	trace				65	1	89
Canned, yellow-fleshed, solids and liquid:									
Syrup pack, heavy:									
Halves or									
Slices...........1 cup	257	52	trace				200	1	79
Halves									
(medium) ......2 halves									
Syrup..........2 tablespoons....	117	24	trace				90	trace	79
Water pack ......1 cup	245	20	trace				75	1	91
Strained or chopped									
(baby food) ......1 ounce	28	6	trace				25	trace	78
Dried:									
Uncooked ....1 cup	160	109	1				420	5	25
Cooked, unsweetened, 10-12 halves and 6 tablespoons									
liquid ....1 cup	270	58	1				220	3	77
Frozen:									
Carton, 12 ounces, not thawed ....1 carton............	340	77	trace				300	1	76

NUTRITIVE VALUES OF THE EDIBLE PART OF FOOD

Food, approximate measure, and weight (in grams)		Carbo-hydrate	Fat (total lipid)	Fatty Acids			Food Energy	Pro-tein	Water
				Satu-rated (total)	Unsaturated Oleic	Linoleic			
	grams	grams	grams	grams	grams	grams	Calories	grams	Percent
Can, 16 ounces, not thawed ....1 can............	454	103	trace				400	2	76
Peach nectar, canned ....1 cup	250	31	trace				120	trace	87
Pears:									
Raw, 3-inch x 2-1/2-inch diameter[1].........1 pear	182	25	1				100	1	83
Canned, solids and liquid:									
Syrup pack, heavy:									
Halves or									
Slices ....1 cup	255	50	1				195	1	80
Halves (medium)..2 halves	117	23	trace				90	trace	80
Syrup ....2 tablespoons....	243	20	trace				80	trace	91
Water pack ....1 cup									
Strained or chopped									
(baby food) ....1 ounce	28	5	trace				20	trace	82
Pear nectar, canned...1 cup	250	33	trace				130	1	86
Persimmons, Japanese or kaki, raw, seedless, 2 1/2-inch									
diameter[1].........1 persimmon.....	125	20	trace				75	1	79
Pineapple:									
Raw, diced.........1 cup	140	19	trace				75	1	85
Canned, heavy syrup pack, solids and liquid:									
Crushed ....1 cup	260	50	trace				195	1	80

[1]-Measure and weight apply to entire vegetable or fruit including parts not usually eaten.

NUTRITIVE VALUES OF THE EDIBLE PART OF FOOD

Food, approximate measure, and weight (in grams)		Carbohydrate	Fat (total lipid)	Fatty Acids Saturated (total)	Unsaturated Oleic	Linoleic	Food Energy	Protein	Water
	grams	grams	grams	grams	grams	grams	Calories	grams	Percent
Sliced, slices and juice........2 small or 1 large 2 tablespoons....	122	24	trace				90	trace	80
Pineapple juice, canned............1 cup	249	34	trace				135	1	86
Plums, all except prunes: Raw, 2-inch diameter, about 2 ounces[1]......1 plum............	60	7	trace				25	trace	87
Plums (without pits) and juice............3 plums 2 tablespoons....	122	26	trace				100	trace	77
Prunes, dried, "softenized," medium: Uncooked[1]............4 prunes	32	18	trace				70	1	28
Cooked, unsweetened, 17-18 prunes and 1/3 cup liquid[1]............1 cup	270	78	1				295	2	66
Prunes with tapioca, canned, strained or junior (baby food)............1 ounce	28	6	trace				200	1	80
Prune juice, canned...............1 cup	256	49	trace				200	1	80
Raisins, dried............1 cup	160	124	trace				460	4	18
Raspberries, red: Raw...............1 cup	123	17	1				70	1	84

[1]-Measure and weight apply to entire vegetable or fruit including parts not usually eaten.

NUTRITIVE VALUES OF THE EDIBLE PART OF FOOD

Food, approximate measure, and weight (in grams)	grams	Carbo-hydrate grams	Fat (total lipid) grams	Fatty Acids Saturated (total) grams	Unsaturated Oleic grams	Unsaturated Linoleic grams	Food Energy Calories	Protein grams	Water Percent
Frozen, 10-ounce carton, not thawed............1 carton	284	70	1				275	2	74
Rhubarb, cooked, sugar added............1 cup	272	98	trace				385	1	63
Strawberries:									
Raw, capped............1 cup	149	13	1				55	1	90
Frozen, 10-ounce carton, not thawed............1 carton	284	79	1				310	1	71
Frozen, 16-ounce can, not thawed............1 can	454	126	1				495	2	71
Tangerines, raw, medium, 2 1/2-inch diameter, about 4 per pound[1]............1 tangerine	114	10	trace				40	1	87
Tangerine juice: Canned, unsweetened............1 cup	248	25	trace				105	1	89
Frozen concentrate: Undiluted, can, 6 fluid ounces............1 can	210	80	1				340	4	58
Diluted with 3 parts water, by volume............1 cup	248	27	trace				115	1	88

[1]-Measure and weight apply to entire vegetable or fruit including parts not usually eaten.

NUTRITIVE VALUES OF THE EDIBLE PART OF FOOD

Food, approximate measure, and weight (in grams)	grams	Carbo-hy-drate grams	Fat (total lipid) grams	Fatty Acids Saturated (total) grams	Oleic grams	Linoleic grams	Food Energy Calories	Protein grams	Water Percent
Watermelon, raw, wedge, 4 inches by 8 inches (1/16 of 10 by 16-inch melon, about 2 pounds with rind)[1]...1 wedge	925	27	1				115	2	93
GRAIN PRODUCTS									
Barley, pearled, light, uncooked ...1 cup	203	160	2	trace	1	1	710	17	11
Biscuits, baking powder with enriched flour, 2 1/2-inch diameter ...1 biscuit	38	17	6	2	3	1	140	3	27
Bran flakes (40 percent bran) added thiamine ...1 ounce	28	23	1				85	3	3
Breads:									
Boston brown bread Slice, 3 inches x 3/4 inch...1 slice	48	22	1				100	3	45
Cracked-wheat bread: Loaf, 1-pound 20 slices...1 loaf	454	236	10	2	5	2	1,190	39	35
Slice...1 slice	23	12	1				60	2	35

[1]-Measure and weight apply to entire vegetable or fruit including parts not usually eaten.

NUTRITIVE VALUES OF THE EDIBLE PART OF FOOD

Food, approximate measure, and weight (in grams)	grams	Carbo-hy-drate grams	Fat (total lipid) grams	Fatty Acids Satu-rated (total) grams	Fatty Acids Unsatu-rated Oleic grams	Fatty Acids Unsatu-rated Lino-leic grams	Food Energy Calo-ries	Pro-tein grams	Water Per-cent
French or Vienna bread:									
Enriched, 1-pound loaf ....1 loaf	454	251	14	3	8	2	1,315	41	31
Unenriched, 1-pound loaf ....1 loaf	454	251	14	3	8	2	1,315	41	31
Italian bread:									
Enriched, 1-pound loaf............1 loaf	454	256	4	trace	1	2	1,250	41	32
Unenriched, 1-pound loaf............1 loaf	454	256	4	trace	1	2	1,250	41	32
Raisin bread:									
Loaf, 1-pound............1 loaf	454	243	13	3	8	2	1,190	30	35
Slice............1 slice	23	12	1				60	2	35
Rye bread:									
American, light (1/3 rye, 2/3 wheat):									
Loaf, 1 pound, 20 slices......1 loaf	454	236	5				1,100	41	36
Slice...........1 slice	23	12	trace				55	2	36
Pumpernickel, loaf, 1 pound.........1 loaf	454	241	5				1,115	41	34

NUTRITIVE VALUES OF THE EDIBLE PART OF FOOD

Food, approximate measure, and weight (in grams)	Carbohydrate	Fat (total lipid)	Fatty Acids Saturated (total)	Unsaturated Oleic	Unsaturated Linoleic	Food Energy	Protein	Water
grams	grams	grams	grams	grams	grams	Calories	grams	Percent
White bread, enriched:								
1 to 2 percent nonfat dry milk:								
Loaf, 1-pound								
20 slices.......1 loaf 454	229	15	3	8	2	1,225	39	36
Slice..........1 slice 23	12	1	trace	trace	trace	60	2	36
3 to 4 percent nonfat dry milk:[2]								
Loaf, 1-pound..........1 loaf 454	229	15	3	8	2	1,225	39	36
Slice, 20 per loaf........1 slice 23	12	1	trace	trace	trace	60	2	36
Slice, toasted.....1 slice 20	12	1	trace	trace	trace	60	2	25
Slice, 26 per loaf..........1 slice 17	9	1	trace	trace	trace	45	1	36
5 to 6 percent nonfat dry milk:								
Loaf, 1-pound, 20 slices.......1 loaf 454	228	17	4	10	2	1,245	41	35
Slice..........1 slice 23	12	1	trace	trace	trace	65	2	35

2-When the amount of nonfat dry milk in commercial white bread is unknown, values for bread with 3 to 4 percent nonfat dry milk are suggested.

NUTRITIVE VALUES OF THE EDIBLE PART OF FOOD

Food, approximate measure, and weight (in grams)		Carbohydrate	Fat (total lipid)	Fatty Acids			Food Energy	Protein	Water
				Saturated (total)	Oleic	Linoleic			
	grams	grams	grams	grams	grams	grams	Calories	grams	Percent
White bread, unenriched:									
1 to 2 percent nonfat dry milk:									
Loaf, 1-pound,									
20 slices........1 loaf	454	229	15	3	8	2	1,225	39	36
Slice............1 slice	23	12	1	trace	trace	trace	60	2	36
3 to 4 percent nonfat dry milk:[2]									
Loaf, 1-pound ....1 loaf	454	229	15	3	8	2	1,225	39	36
Slice, 20 per loaf............1 slice	23	12	1	trace	trace	trace	60	2	36
Slice, toasted ....1 slice	20	12	1	trace	trace	trace	60	2	25
Slice, 26 per loaf............1 slice	17	9	1	trace	trace	trace	45	1	36
5 to 6 percent nonfat dry milk:									
Loaf, 1-pound,									
20 slices........1 loaf	454	228	17	4	10	2	1,245	41	35
Slice............1 slice	23	12	1	trace	trace	trace	65	2	35
Whole-wheat bread, made with 2 percent nonfat dry milk:									
Loaf, 1-pound,									
20 slices............1 loaf	454	216	14	3	6	3	1,105	48	36
Slice............1 slice	23	11	1	trace	trace	trace	55	2	36

[2]-When the amount of nonfat dry milk in commercial white bread is unknown, values for bread with 3 to 4 percent nonfat dry milk are suggested.

NUTRITVE VALUES OF THE EDIBLE PART OF FOOD

Food, approximate measure, and weight (in grams)	grams	Carbohydrate grams	Fat (total lipid) grams	Fatty Acids Saturated (total) grams	Unsaturated Oleic grams	Linoleic grams	Food Energy Calories	Protein grams	Water Percent
Slice, toasted...........1 slice............	19	11	1	trace	trace	trace	55	2	24
Bread crumbs, dry grated ....1 cup	88	65	4	1	2	1	345	11	6
Cakes:[3]									
Angel food cake, sector, 2-inch (1/12 of 8-inch diameter cake)............1 sector	40	24	trace				110	3	32
Chocolate cake, chocolate icing; sector, 2-inch (1/16 of 10-inch diameter layer cake)............1 sector	120	67	20	8	10	1	445	5	22
Fruitcake, dark (made with enriched flour); piece, 2 inches by 2 inches by 1/2 inch ....1 piece............	30	18	5	1	3	1	115	1	18
Gingerbread (made with enriched flour); piece, 2 inches by 2 inches by 2 inches............1 piece............	55	29	6	1	4	trace	175	2	31

3-Unenriched cake flour and vegetable cooking fat used unless otherwise specified.

198

NUTRITIVE VALUES OF THE EDIBLE PART OF FOOD

Food, approximate measure, and weight (in grams)	grams	Carbo-hydrate grams	Fat (total lipid) grams	Fatty Acids Satu-rated (total) grams	Unsaturated Oleic grams	Unsaturated Lino-leic grams	Food Energy Calories	Pro-tein grams	Water Per-cent
Plain cake and cupcakes without icing:									
Piece, 3 inches by 2 inches by 1 1/2 inches ...1 piece	55	31	8	2	5	1	200	2	24
Cupcake, 2 3/4-inch diameter ...1 cupcake	40	22	6	1	3	trace	145	2	24
Plain cake and cupcakes, with chocolate icing:									
Sector, 2-inch (1/16 of 10-inch layer cake)...1 sector	100	59	14	5	7	1	370	4	21
Cupcake, 2 3/4-inch diameter ...1 cupcake	50	30	7	2	4	trace	185	2	21
Pound cake, old-fashioned (equal weights flour, sugar, fat, eggs); Slice, 2 3/4 inches by 3 inches by 5/8 inch ...1 slice	30	14	9	2	5	1	140	2	17
Sponge cake; sector, 2-inch (1/12 of 8-inch diameter cake) ...1 sector	40	22	2	1	1	trace	120	3	32
Cookies:									
Plain and assorted, 3-inch diameter ...1 cookie	25	18	5				120	1	3
Fig bars, small ...1 fig bar	16	12	1				55	1	14

NUTRITIVE VALUES OF THE EDIBLE PART OF FOOD

Food, approximate measure, and weight (in grams)		Carbohydrate	Fat (total lipid)	Fatty Acids			Food Energy	Protein	Water
				Saturated (total)	Unsaturated Oleic	Unsaturated Linoleic			
	grams	grams	grams	grams	grams	grams	Calories	grams	Percent
Corn, rice and wheat flakes, mixed, added nutrients............1 ounce	28	24	trace				110	2	3
Cornflakes, added nutrients:									
Plain..................1 ounce	28	24	trace				110	2	4
Sugar-covered........1 ounce	28	26	trace				110	1	2
Corn grits, degermed, cooked:									
Enriched............1 cup	242	27	trace				120	3	87
Unenriched..........1 cup	242	27	trace				120	3	87
Cornmeal, white or yellow, dry:									
Whole ground, unbolted............1 cup	118	87	5	1	2	2	420	11	12
Degermed, enriched............1 cup	145	114	2	trace	1	1	525	11	12
Corn muffins, made with enriched degermed cornmeal and enriched flour; muffin 2 3/4-inch diameter..1 muffin	48	23	5	2	2	trace	150	3	33
Corn, puffed, presweetened, added nutrients ......1 ounce	28	26	trace				110	1	5
Corn, shredded, added nutrients..............1 ounce	28	25	trace				110	2	3
Crackers:									
Graham, plain ....4 small or 2 medium.........	14	10	1				55	1	6

NUTRITIVE VALUES OF THE EDIBLE PART OF FOOD

Food, approximate measure, and weight (in grams)		Carbo-hydrate	Fat (total lipid)	Fatty Acids			Food Energy	Pro-tein	Water
				Satu-rated (total)	Unsaturated				
					Oleic	Lino-leic			
	grams	grams	grams	grams	grams	grams	Calories	grams	Percent
Saltines, 2 inches square ....2 crackers	8	6	1				35	1	4
Soda:									
Cracker, 2 1/2 inches square ......2 crackers	11	8	1	trace	1	trace	50	1	4
Oyster crackers.......10 crackers......	10	7	1	trace	1	trace	45	1	4
Cracker meal...........1 tablespoon......	10	7	1	trace	1	trace	45	1	6
Doughnuts, cake type...1 doughnut......	32	16	6	1	4	trace	125	1	24
Farina, regular, enriched, cooked ....1 cup	238	21	trace				100	3	90
Macaroni, cooked:									
Enriched:									
Cooked, firm stage (8 to 10 minutes; undergoes additional cooking in a food mixture) ....1 cup	130	39	1				190	6	64
Cooked until tender ....1 cup	140	32	1				155	5	72
Unenriched:									
Cooked, firm stage (8 to 10 minutes; undergoes additional cooking in a food mixture) ....1 cup	130	39	1				190	6	64
Cooked until tender ....1 cup	140	32	1				155	5	72

NUTRITIVE VALUES OF THE EDIBLE PART OF FOOD

Food, approximate measure, and weight (in grams)		Carbo-hy-drate	Fat (total lipid)	Fatty Acids			Food Energy	Pro-tein	Water
				Satu-rated (total)	Unsaturated				
					Oleic	Lino-leic			
	grams	grams	grams	grams	grams	grams	Calo-ries	grams	Per-cent
Macaroni (enriched) and cheese, baked..........1 cup	220	44	24	11	10	1	470	18	58
Muffins, with enriched white flour; muffin 2 3/4-inch diameter ....1 muffin	48	20	5	1	3	trace	140	4	38
Noodles (egg noodles), cooked:									
Enriched ....1 cup	160	37	2	1	1	trace	200	7	70
Unenriched ....1 cup	160	37	2	1	1	trace	200	7	70
Oats (with or without corn) puffed, added nutrient ....1 ounce	28	21	2	trace	1	1	115	3	3
Oatmeal or rolled oats, regular or quick-cooking, cooked ....1 cup	236	23	2	trace	1	1	130	5	86
Pancakes (griddlecakes), 4-inch diameter:									
Wheat, enriched flour (home recipe)..........1 cake	27	9	2	trace	1	trace	60	2	50
Buckwheat (buckwheat pancake mix, made with egg and milk)..........1 cake	27	6	2	1	1	trace	55	2	58
Piecrust, plain, baked: Enriched flour: Lower crust, 9-inch shell..........1 crust	135	59	45	10	29	3	675	8	15

NUTRITIVE VALUES OF THE EDIBLE PART OF FOOD

Food, approximate measure, and weight (in grams)	grams	Carbo-hydrate grams	Fat (total lipid) grams	Fatty Acids Satu-rated (total) grams	Unsaturated Oleic grams	Unsaturated Lino-leic grams	Food Energy Calories	Pro-tein grams	Water Per-cent
Double crust, 9-inch pie............1 double crust...	270	118	90	21	58	7	1,350	16	15
Pies (piecrust made with unenriched flour); sector, 4-inch, 1/7 of 9-inch pie:									
Apple............1 sector	135	51	15	4	9	1	345	3	48
Cherry............1 sector	135	52	15	4	10	1	355	4	47
Custard ....1 sector	130	30	14	5	8	1	280	8	58
Lemon Meringue .1 sector	120	45	12	4	7	1	305	4	47
Mince ....1 sector	135	56	16	4	10	1	365	3	43
Pumpkin............1 sector	130	32	15	5	7	1	275	5	59
Pizza (cheese); 5 1/2-inch sector; 1/8 of 14-inch diameter pie ....1 sector	75	27	6	2	3	trace	185	7	45
Popcorn, popped, with added oil and salt.........1 cup	14	8	3	2	trace	trace	65	1	3
Pretzels, small stick............5 sticks..........	4	4	trace				20	trace	8
Rice, white (fully milled or polished), enriched, cooked:									
Common commercial varieties, all types............1 cup	168	41	trace				185	3	73
Long grain, parboiled ....1 cup	176	41	trace				185	4	73

NUTRITIVE VALUES OF THE EDIBLE PART OF FOOD

Food, approximate measure, and weight (in grams)		Carbohydrate	Fat (total lipid)	Fatty Acids			Food Energy	Protein	Water
				Saturated (total)	Unsaturated				
					Oleic	Linoleic			
	grams	grams	grams	grams	grams	grams	Calories	grams	Percent
Rice, puffed, added nutrients (without salt)............1 cup	14	13	trace				55	1	4
Rice flakes, added nutrients...............1 cup	30	26	trace				115	2	3
Rolls:									
Plain, pan; 12 per 16 ounces:									
Enriched............1 roll	38	20	2	trace	1	trace	115	3	31
Unenriched.........1 roll	38	20	2	trace	1	trace	115	3	31
Hard, round; 12 per 22 ounces............1 roll	52	31	2	trace	1	trace	160	5	25
Sweet, pan; 12 per 18 ounces............1 roll	43	21	4	1	2	trace	135	4	32
Rye wafers, whole-grain, 1 7/8 inches by 3 1/2 inches............2 wafers	13	10	trace				45	2	6
Spaghetti with meatballs in tomato sauce (home recipe)............1 cup	250	37	9	2	5	1	260	9	77
Waffles, with enriched flour, 1/2 inch by 4 1/2 inches by 5 1/2 inches............1 waffle	75	28	7	2	4	1	210	7	41
Wheat, puffed: With added nutrients (without salt)......1 ounce	28	22	trace				105	4	3

204

NUTRITIVE VALUES OF THE EDIBLE PART OF FOOD

Food, approximate measure, and weight (in grams)		Carbo-hy-drate	Fat (total lipid)	Fatty Acids Saturated (total)	Unsaturated Oleic	Unsaturated Lino-leic	Food Energy	Pro-tein	Water
	grams	grams	grams	grams	grams	grams	Calo-ries	grams	Per-cent
With added nutrients, with sugar and honey.........1 ounce	28	25	1				105	2	3
Wheat, rolled: cooked.............1 cup	235	40	1				100	3	7
Wheat, shredded, plain (long, round, or bite-size).........1 ounce	28	23	1				100	3	7
Wheat and malted barley flakes, with added nutrients.........1 ounce	28	23	trace				100	3	4
Wheat flours: Whole-wheat, from hard wheats, stirred.........1 cup	120	85	2	trace	1	1	400	16	12
All-purpose or family flour: Enriched, sifted..........1 cup	110	84	1	trace	trace	trace	400	12	12
Unenriched, sifted..........1 cup	110	84	1	trace	trace	trace	400	12	12
Self-rising, enriched..........1 cup	110	82	1	trace	trace	trace	385	1	11
Cake or pastry flour, sifted..........1 cup	100	79	1	trace	trace	trace	365	8	12
Wheat germ, crude, commercially milled..........1 cup	68	32	7	1	2	4	245	18	11

NUTRITIVE VALUES OF THE EDIBLE PART OF FOOD

Food, approximate measure, and weight (in grams)	grams	Carbo-hy-drate grams	Fat (total lipid) grams	Fatty Acids Satu-rated (total) grams	Unsaturated Oleic grams	Unsaturated Lino-leic grams	Food Energy Calo-ries	Pro-tein grams	Water Per-cent
MATURE DRY BEANS AND PEAS, NUTS, PEANUTS: RELATED PRODUCTS									
Almonds,									
shelled............1 cup	142	28	77	6	52	15	850	26	5
Beans, dry:									
Common varieties, such as									
Great Northern, navy, and									
others, canned:									
Red ....1 cup	256	42	1				230	15	76
White, with tomato sauce:									
with pork......1 cup	261	50	7	3	3	1	320	16	71
without pork...1 cup	261	60	1				310	16	68
Lima,									
cooked ....1 cup	192	48	1				260	16	64
Brazil nuts ....1 cup	140	24	94	19	45	24	915	20	5
Cashew nuts,									
roasted ....1 cup	135	40	62	10	43	4	760	23	5
Coconut:									
Fresh, shredded......1 cup	97	9	34	29	2	trace	335	3	51
Dried, shredded,									
sweetened.........1 cup	62	33	24	21	2	trace	340	2	3
Cowpeas or blackeye peas,									
dried, cooked........1 cup	248	34	1				190	13	80

NUTRITIVE VALUES OF THE EDIBLE PART OF FOOD

Food, approximate measure, and weight (in grams)	Carbohydrate	Fat (total lipid)	Fatty Acids Saturated (total)	Fatty Acids Unsaturated Oleic	Fatty Acids Unsaturated Linoleic	Food Energy	Protein	Water
grams	grams	grams	grams	grams	grams	Calories	grams	Percent
Peanuts, roasted, salted:								
Halves............1 cup 144	27	72	16	31	21	840	37	2
Chopped.........1 tablespoon 9	2	4	1	2	1	55	2	2
Peanut butter.........1 tablespoon 16	3	8	2	4	2	95	4	2
Peas, split, dry, cooked ....1 cup 250	52	1				290	20	70
Pecans:								
Halves............1 cup 108	16	77	5	48	15	740	10	3
Chopped.........1 tablespoon 7.5	1	5	trace	3	1	50	1	3
Walnuts, shelled:								
Black or native, chopped.........1 cup 126	19	75	4	26	36	790	26	3
English or Persian:								
Halves............1 cup 100	16	64	4	10	40	650	15	4
Chopped.........1 tablespoon 8	1	5	trace	1	3	50	1	4
MEAT, POULTRY, FISH, SHELLFISH: RELATED PRODUCTS								
Bacon, broiled or fried, crisp ....2 slices 16	1	8	3	4	1	100	5	8
Beef, trimmed to retail basis,[4] cooked:								

4.-Outer layer of fat on the cut was removed to within approximately 1/2 inch of the lean. Deposits of fat within the cut were not removed.

NUTRITIVE VALUES OF THE EDIBLE PART OF FOOD

Food, approximate measure, and weight (in grams)	Carbo-hy-drate	Fat (total lipid)	Fatty Acids Satu-rated (total)	Fatty Acids Unsaturated Oleic	Fatty Acids Unsaturated Lino-leic	Food Energy	Pro-tein	Water
grams	grams	grams	grams	grams	grams	Calo-ries	grams	Per-cent
Cuts braised, simmered, or pot-roasted:								
Lean and fat......3 ounces 85	0	16	8	7	trace	245	23	53
Lean only ....2.5 ounces......... 72	0	5	2	2	trace	140	22	62
Hamburger (ground beef), broiled:								
Lean......3 ounces 85	0	10	5	4	trace	185	23	60
Regular......3 ounces 85	0	17	8	8	trace	245	21	54
Roast, oven-cooked, no liquid added:								
Relatively fat, such as rib:								
Lean and fat......3 ounces......... 85	0	34	15	16	1	375	17	40
Lean only ....1.8 ounces......... 51	0	7	3	3	trace	125	14	57
Relatively lean, such as heel of round:								
Lean and fat......3 ounces......... 85	0	7	3	3	trace	165	25	62
Lean only ....2.7 ounces......... 78	0	3	1	1	trace	125	24	65
Steak, broiled:								
Relatively fat, such as sirloin:								
Lean and fat......3 ounces......... 85	0	27	13	12	1	330	20	44
Lean only ....2 ounces......... 56	0	4	2	2	trace	115	18	59
Relatively lean, such as round:								
Lean and fat......3 ounces......... 85	0	13	6	6	trace	220	24	55
Lean only ....2.4 ounces......... 68	0	4	2	2	trace	130	21	61
Beef, canned:								
Corned beef.........3 ounces......... 85	0	10	5	4	trace	185	22	59
Corned beef hash....3 ounces......... 85	9	10	5	4	trace	155	7	67

208

NUTRITIVE VALUES OF THE EDIBLE PART OF FOOD

Food, approximate measure, and weight (in grams)		Carbohydrate	Fat (total lipid)	Fatty Acids Saturated (total)	Unsaturated Oleic	Linoleic	Food Energy	Protein	Water
	grams	grams	grams	grams	grams	grams	Calories	grams	Percent
Beef, dried or chipped ...2 ounces	57	0	4	2	2	trace	115	19	48
Beef and vegetable stew ...1 cup	235	15	10	5	4	trace	210	15	82
Beef potpie, baked: Individual pie, 4 1/4-inch diameter, weight before baking about 8 ounces ...1 pie	227	43	33	9	20	2	560	23	55
Chicken, cooked: Flesh only, broiled ...3 ounces	85	0	3	1	1	1	115	20	71
Breast, fried, 1/2 breast: With bone ...3.3 ounces	94	1	5	1	2	1	155	25	58
Flesh and skin only ...2.7 ounces	76	1	5	1	2	1	155	25	58
Drumstick, fried: With bone ...2.1 ounces	59	trace	4	1	2	1	90	12	55
Flesh and skin only ...1.3 ounces	38	trace	4	1	2	1	90	12	55
Chicken, canned, boneless ...3 ounces	85	0	10	3	4	2	170	18	65
Chicken potpie. SEE Poultry potpie.									

NUTRITIVE VALUES OF THE EDIBLE PART OF FOOD

Food, approximate measure, and weight (in grams)		Carbohydrate	Fat (total lipid)	Fatty Acids			Food Energy	Protein	Water
				Saturated (total)	Unsaturated Oleic	Unsaturated Linoleic			
	grams	grams	grams	grams	grams	grams	Calories	grams	Percent
Chili con carne, canned:									
With beans.........1 cup	250	30	15	7	7	trace	335	19	72
Without beans.........1 cup	255	15	38	18	17	1	510	26	67
Heart, beef, lean, braised.........3 ounces	85	1	5	....	....	....	160	27	61
Lamb, trimmed to retail basis,[4] cooked:									
Chop, thick, with bone, broiled.........1 chop,									
4.8 ounces	137	0	33	18	12	1	400	25	47
Lean and fat.....4.0 ounces	112	0	33	18	12	1	400	25	47
Lean only.......2.6 ounces	74	0	6	3	2	trace	140	21	62
Leg, roasted:									
Lean and fat.....3 ounces	85	0	16	9	6	trace	235	22	54
Lean only.......2.5 ounces	71	0	5	3	2	trace	130	20	62
Shoulder, roasted:									
Lean and fat.....3 ounces	85	0	23	13	8	1	285	18	50
Lean only.......2.3 ounces	64	0	6	3	2	trace	130	17	61
Liver, beef, fried.........2 ounces	57	3	6	....	....	....	130	15	57
Pork, cured, cooked:									
Ham, light cure, lean and fat, roasted.........3 ounces	85	0	19	7	8	2	245	18	54

[4]-Outer layer of fat on the cut was removed to within approximately 1/2 inch of the lean. Deposits of fat within the cut were not removed.

NUTRITIVE VALUES OF THE EDIBLE PART OF FOOD

Food, approximate measure, and weight (in grams)		Carbohydrate	Fat (total lipid)	Fatty Acids			Food Energy	Protein	Water
				Saturated (total)	Unsaturated Oleic	Linoleic			
	grams	grams	grams	grams	grams	grams	Calories	grams	Percent
Luncheon meat:									
Boiled ham, sliced ....2 ounces	57	0	10	4	4	1	135	11	59
Canned, spiced or unspiced ....2 ounces	57	1	14	5	6	1	165	8	55
Pork, fresh, trimmed to retail basis,[4] cooked:									
Chop, thick, with bone ....1 chop, 3.5 ounces.........	98	0	21	8	9	2	260	16	42
Lean and fat ......2.3 ounces.........	66	0	21	8	9	2	260	16	42
Lean only ....1.7 ounces.........	48	0	7	2	3	1	130	15	53
Roast, oven-cooked, no liquid added:									
Lean and fat......3 ounces	85	0	24	9	10	2	310	21	46
Lean only ....2.4 ounces.........	68	0	10	3	4	1	175	20	55
Cuts, simmered:									
Lean and fat......3 ounces.........	85	0	26	9	11	2	320	20	46
Lean only ....2.2 ounces.........	63	0	6	2	3	1	135	18	60
Poultry potpie (based on chicken potpie) Individual pie, 4 1/4-inch diameter, weight before baking about 8 ounces ....1 pie	227	42	31	10	15	3	535	23	57

[4]-Outer layer of fat on the cut was removed to within approximately 1/2 inch of the lean. Deposits of fat within the cut were not removed.

NUTRITIVE VALUES OF THE EDIBLE PART OF FOOD

Food, approximate measure, and weight (in grams)		Carbo-hy-drate	Fat (total lipid)	Fatty Acids			Food Energy	Pro-tein	Water
				Satu-rated (total)	Unsaturated				
					Oleic	Lino-leic			
	grams	grams	grams	grams	grams	grams	Calo-ries	grams	Per-cent
Sausage:									
Bologna, slice, 4.1 inch by 0.1 inch ....8 slices	227	2	62				690	27	56
Frankfurter, cooked ....1 frankfurter.....	51	1	14				155	6	58
Pork, links or patty, cooked ....4 ounces...........	113	trace	50	18	21	5	540	21	35
Tongue, beef, braised ....3 ounces	85	trace	14				210	18	61
Turkey potpie. SEE poultry potpie.									
Veal, cooked:									
Cutlet, without bone, broiled ....3 ounces	85	....	9	5	4	trace	185	23	60
Roast, medium fat, medium done; lean and fat...........3 ounces	85	0	14	7	6	trace	230	23	55
Fish and shellfish:									
Bluefish, baked or broiled ....3 ounces	85	0	4				135	22	68
Clams:									
Raw, meat only...3 ounces	85	2	1				65	11	82
Canned, solids and liquid ....3 ounces	85	2	1				45	7	86
Crabmeat, canned ....3 ounces	85	1	2				85	15	77

NUTRITIVE VALUES OF THE EDIBLE PART OF FOOD

Food, approximate measure, and weight (in grams)		Carbohydrate	Fat (total lipid)	Fatty Acids			Food Energy	Protein	Water
				Saturated (total)	Unsaturated Oleic	Linoleic			
	grams	grams	grams	grams	grams	grams	Calories	grams	Percent
Fish sticks, breaded, cooked, frozen; stick 3.8 inches x 1.0 inch x 0.5 inch............10 sticks or 8-ounce package..........	227	15	20	5	4	10	400	38	66
Haddock, fried ....3 ounces..........	85	5	5	1	3	trace	140	17	66
Mackerel: Broiled, Atlantic..........3 ounces	85	0	13				200	19	62
Canned, Pacific, solids and liquid[5].......3 ounces	85	0	9				155	18	66
Ocean perch, breaded (egg and bread crumbs), fried.......3 ounces	85	6	11				195	16	59
Oysters, meat only: Raw, 13-19 medium selects................1 cup	240	8	4				160	20	85
Stew, 1 part oysters to 3 parts milk by volume, 3-4 oysters............1 cup	230	11	12				200	11	84
Salmon, pink, canned............3 ounces	85	0	5	1	1	trace	120	17	71
Sardines, Atlantic, canned in oil, drained solids ....3 ounces	85	0	9				175	20	62

5-Vitamin values based on drained solids.

NUTRITIVE VALUES OF THE EDIBLE PART OF FOOD

Food, approximate measure, and weight (in grams)	grams	Carbo-hy-drate grams	Fat (total lipid) grams	Fatty Acids Satu-rated (total) grams	Unsaturated Oleic grams	Linoleic grams	Food Energy Calories	Protein grams	Water Percent
Shad, baked ....3 ounces.........	85	0	10				170	20	64
Swordfish, broiled with butter or margarine ....3 ounces.........	85	0	5				150	24	65
Tuna, canned in oil, drained solids ....3 ounces.........	85	0	7				170	24	61
MILK, CREAM, CHEESE: RELATED PRODUCTS									
Milk, cow's:									
Fluid, whole (3.5% fat).............1 cup	244	12	9	5	3	trace	160	9	87
Fluid, nonfat (skim).............1 cup	246	13	trace				90	9	90
Buttermilk, cultured, from skim milk ...1 cup	246	13	trace				90	9	90
Evaporated, unsweetened, undiluted ....1 cup	252	24	20	11	7	1	245	18	74
Condensed, sweetened, undiluted ....1 cup	306	166	27	15	9	1	980	25	27
Dry, whole.............1 cup	103	39	28	16	9	1	515	27	2
Dry, nonfat, instant.............1 cup	70	36	trace				250	25	3

NUTRITIVE VALUES OF THE EDIBLE PART OF FOOD

Food, approximate measure, and weight (in grams)		Carbohydrate	Fat (total lipid)	Fatty Acids			Food Energy	Protein	Water
				Saturated (total)	Unsaturated				
					Oleic	Linoleic			
	grams	grams	grams	grams	grams	grams	Calories	grams	Percent
Milk, goat's:									
Fluid, whole........1 cup	244	11	10	6	2	trace	165	8	88
Cream:									
Half-and-half (cream and milk)........1 cup	242	11	28	16	9	1	325	8	80
1 tablespoon......	15	1	2	1	1	trace	20	trace	80
Light, coffee or table........1 cup	240	10	49	27	16	1	505	7	72
1 tablespoon......	15	1	3	2	1	trace	30	trace	72
Whipping, unwhipped (volume about double when whipped):									
Light........1 cup	239	9	75	41	25	2	715	6	62
1 tablespoon......	15	1	5	3	2	trace	45	trace	62
Heavy........1 cup	238	7	89	49	29	3	840	5	57
1 tablespoon......	15	trace	6	3	2	trace	55	trace	57
Cheese:									
Blue or Roquefort type........1 ounce	28	1	9	5	3	trace	105	6	40
Cheddar or American:									
Ungrated........1-inch cube	17	trace	5	3	2	trace	70	4	37
Grated........1 cup	112	2	36	20	12	1	445	28	37
1 tablespoon......	7	trace	2	1	1	trace	30	2	37
Cheddar, process....1 ounce	28	1	9	5	3	trace	105	7	40
Cheese foods, Cheddar........1 ounce	28	2	7	4	2	trace	90	6	43

NUTRITIVE VALUES OF THE EDIBLE PART OF FOOD

Food, approximate measure, and weight (in grams)	grams	Carbo-hydrate grams	Fat (total lipid) grams	Fatty Acids Satu-rated (total) grams	Unsatu-rated Oleic grams	Lino-leic grams	Food Energy Calories	Pro-tein grams	Water Per-cent
Cottage cheese, from skim milk:									
Creamed .... 1 cup	225	7	9	5	3	trace	240	31	78
1 ounce	28	1	1	1	trace	trace	30	4	78
Uncreamed ...... 1 cup	225	6	1	trace	trace	trace	195	38	79
1 ounce	28	1	trace				25	5	79
Cream cheese .... 1 ounce	28	1	11	6	4	trace	105	2	51
1 tablespoon	15	trace	6	3	2	trace	55	1	51
Swiss (domestic) .... 1 ounce	28	1	8	4	3	trace	105	8	39
Milk beverages:									
Cocoa .... 1 cup	242	26	11	6	4	trace	235	9	79
Chocolate-flavored milk drink (made with skim milk) .... 1 cup	250	27	6	3	2	trace	190	8	83
Malted milk .... 1 cup	270	32	12				280	13	78
Milk desserts:									
Cornstarch pudding, plain (blanc mange) .... 1 cup	248	39	10	5	3	trace	275	9	76
Custard, baked ...... 1 cup	248	28	14	6	5	1	285	13	77
Ice cream, plain, factory packed: Slice or cut brick, 1/8 of quart brick .... 1 slice or cut brick	71	15	9	5	3	trace	145	3	62

NUTRITIVE VALUES OF THE EDIBLE PART OF FOOD

Food, approximate measure, and weight (in grams)		Carbohydrate	Fat (total lipid)	Fatty Acids			Food Energy	Protein	Water
				Saturated (total)	Unsaturated Oleic	Linoleic			
	grams	grams	grams	grams	grams	grams	Calories	grams	Percent
Container.........3 1/2 fluid ounces.........	62	13	8	4	3	trace	130	2	62
Container.........8 fluid ounces ...	142	29	18	10	6	1	295	6	62
Ice milk........1 cup............	187	42	10	6	3	trace	285	9	67
Yogurt, from partially skim milk ....1 cup	246	13	4	2	1	trace	120	8	89
EGGS									
Eggs, large, 24 ounces per dozen:									
Raw:									
Whole, without shell..........1 egg.............	50	trace	6	2	3	trace	80	6	74
White of egg...1 white...........	33	trace	trace				15	4	88
Yolk of egg ....1 yolk	17	trace	5	2	2	trace	60	3	51
Cooked:									
Boiled, shell removed ....2 eggs.............	100	1	12	4	5	1	160	12	74
Scrambled with milk and fat ...1 egg.............	64	1	8	3	3	trace	110	7	72
SUGARS, SWEETS									
Candy:									
Caramels ....1 ounce	28	22	3	2	1	trace	115	1	8

NUTRITIVE VALUES OF THE EDIBLE PART OF FOOD

Food, approximate measure, and weight (in grams)	weight (grams)	Carbo-hydrate (grams)	Fat (total lipid) (grams)	Fatty Acids Saturated (total) (grams)	Fatty Acids Unsaturated Oleic (grams)	Fatty Acids Unsaturated Linoleic (grams)	Food Energy (Calories)	Protein (grams)	Water (Percent)
Chocolate, milk,									
plain ....1 ounce	28	16	9	5	3	trace	150	2	1
Fudge, plain ....1 ounce	28	21	3	2	1	trace	115	1	8
Hard candy ....1 ounce	28	28	trace				110	0	1
Marshmallows ....1 ounce	28	23	trace				90	1	17
Chocolate syrup,									
thin type ....1 tablespoon	20	13	trace	trace	trace	trace	50	trace	32
Honey, strained or									
extracted ....1 tablespoon.....	21	17	0				65	trace	17
Jams and preserves ......1 tablespoon.....	20	14	trace				55	trace	29
Jellies ....1 tablespoon.....	20	14	trace				55	trace	29
Molasses, cane: Light (first									
extraction) ....1 tablespoon.....	20	13					50		24
Blackstrap (third									
extraction) ....1 tablespoon.....	20	11					45		24
Syrup, table blends (chiefly corn,									
light and dark) ....1 tablespoon.....	20	15	0				60	0	24
Sugars (cane or beet):									
Granulated............1 cup	200	199	0				770	0	trace
1 tablespoon......	12	12	0				45	0	trace
Lump 1 1/8 inches by 3/4 inch									
by 3/8 inch ....1 lump	6	6	0				25	0	trace
Powdered, stirred before									
measuring ....1 cup	128	127	0				495	0	trace
1 tablespoon......	8	8	0				30	0	trace

NUTRITIVE VALUES OF THE EDIBLE PART OF FOOD

Food, approximate measure, and weight (in grams)		Carbo-hy-drate	Fat (total lipid)	Fatty Acids			Food Energy	Pro-tein	Water
				Satu-rated (total)	Unsaturated Oleic	Linoleic			
	grams	grams	grams	grams	grams	grams	Calo-ries	grams	Per-cent
Brown, firm-packed ....1 cup	220	212	0				820	0	2
1 tablespoon	14	13	0				50	0	2
VEGETABLE AND VEGETABLE PRODUCTS									
Asparagus:									
Cooked, cut spears ..1 cup	175	6	trace				35	4	94
Canned spears, medium:									
Green............6 spears	96	3	trace				20	2	92
Bleached ....6 spears	96	4	trace				20	2	92
Beans:									
Lima, immature cooked ....1 cup	160	32	1				180	1	71
Snap green:									
Cooked:									
In small amount of water, short time............1 cup	125	7	trace				30	2	92
In large amount of water, long time............1 cup	125	7	trace				30	2	92
Canned:									
Solids and liquid ....1 cup	239	10	trace				45	2	94

NUTRITIVE VALUES OF THE EDIBLE PART OF FOOD

Food, approximate measure, and weight (in grams)	grams	Carbo-hy-drate grams	Fat (total lipid) grams	Fatty Acids Satu-rated (total) grams	Unsatu-rated Oleic grams	Unsatu-rated Lino-leic grams	Food Energy Calories	Pro-tein grams	Water Per-cent
Strained or chopped (baby food) ....1 ounce	28	1	trace				5	trace	92
Bean sprouts. SEE sprouts.									
Beets, cooked, diced....1 cup	165	12	trace				50	2	91
Broccoli spears, cooked ....1 cup	150	7	trace				40	5	91
Brussels sprouts, cooked ....1 cup	130	8	1				45	5	88
Cabbage:									
Raw:									
Finely shredded...1 cup	100	5	trace				25	1	92
Coleslaw.............1 cup	120	9	9	2	2	5	120	1	83
Cooked:									
In small amount of water, short time ....1 cup	170	7	trace				35	2	94
In large amount of water, long time ....1 cup	170	7	trace				30	2	94
Cabbage, celery or Chinese:									
Raw, leaves and stalk, 1-inch pieces.........1 cup	100	3	trace				15	1	95
Cabbage, spoon (or Bok Choy), cooked ....1 cup	150	4	trace				20	2	95
Carrots:									
Raw:									
Whole, 5 1/2 inches by 1 inch, (25 thin strips) ...1 carrot...........	50	5	trace				20	1	88

NUTRITIVE VALUES OF THE EDIBLE PART OF FOOD

Food, approximate measure, and weight (in grams)		Carbo-hy-drate	Fat (total lipid)	Fatty Acids Saturated (total)	Unsaturated Oleic	Unsaturated Linoleic	Food Energy	Pro-tein	Water
	grams	grams	grams	grams	grams	grams	Calo-ries	grams	Per-cent
Grated ....1 cup	110	11	trace				45	1	88
Cooked, diced....1 cup	145	10	trace				45	1	91
Canned, strained or chopped (baby food)........1 ounce	28	2	trace				10	trace	92
Cauliflower, cooked, flowerbuds ....1 cup	120	5	trace				25	3	92
Celery:									
Stalk, large outer, 8 inches by about 1 1/2 inches, at root end ....1 stalk	40	2	trace				5	trace	94
Pieces, diced ...1 cup	100	4	trace				15	1	94
Collards, cooked ...1 cup	190	9	1				55	5	91
Corn, sweet:									
Cooked, ear 5 inches by 1 3/4 inches[1].........1 ear..........	140	16	1				70	3	74
Canned, solids and liquid..............1 cup	256	40	2				170	5	81
Cowpeas, cooked, immature seeds...........1 cup	160	29	1				175	13	72
Cucumbers, 10-ounce; 7 1/2 inches by about 2 inches:									
Raw, pared ....1 cucumber	207	7	trace				30	1	96

[1]-Measure and weight apply to entire vegetable or fruit including parts not usually eaten.

NUTRITIVE VALUES OF THE EDIBLE PART OF FOOD

Food, approximate measure, and weight (in grams)	Carbohydrate	Fat (total lipid)	Saturated (total)	Fatty Acids Unsaturated Oleic	Fatty Acids Unsaturated Linoleic	Food Energy	Protein	Water
	grams	grams	grams	grams	grams	grams	Calories	grams	Percent
Raw, pared, center slice 1/8-inch thick ....6 slices	50	2	trace				5	trace	96
Dandelion greens cooked ....1 cup	180	12	1				60	4	90
Endive, curly (including escarole) ....2 ounces	57	2	trace				10	1	93
Kale, leaves including stems, cooked ....1 cup	110	4	1				30	4	91
Lettuce, raw: Butterhead, as Boston types; head, 4-inch diameter ....1 head	120	6	trace				30	3	95
Crisphead, as Iceberg; head; 4 3/4-inch diameter ....1 head	454	13	trace				60	4	96
Looseleaf, or bunching varieties, leaves ....2 large	50	2	trace				10	1	94
Mushrooms, canned, solids and liquid ....1 cup	244	6	trace				40	5	93
Mustard greens, cooked ....1 cup	140	6	1				35	3	93
Okra, cooked, pod 3 inches by 5/8 inch............8 pods	85	5	trace				25	2	91

NUTRITIVE VALUES OF THE EDIBLE PART OF FOOD

Food, approximate measure, and weight (in grams)		Carbo-hy-drate	Fat (total lipid)	Fatty Acids Saturated (total)	Fatty Acids Unsaturated Oleic	Fatty Acids Unsaturated Linoleic	Food Energy	Pro-tein	Water
	grams	grams	grams	grams	grams	grams	Calories	grams	Percent
Onions:									
Mature:									
Raw, onion 2 1/2-inch diameter..........1 onion	110	10	trace				40	2	89
Cooked..........1 cup	210	14	trace				60	3	92
Young green, small without tops..........6 onions	50	5	trace				20	1	88
Parsley, raw, chopped..........1 tablespoon	3.5	trace	trace				1	trace	85
Parsnips, cooked..........1 cup	155	23	1				100	2	82
Peas, green:									
Cooked..........1 cup	160	19	1				115	9	82
Canned, solids and liquid..........1 cup	249	31	1				165	9	83
Canned, strained (baby food)..........1 ounce	28	3	trace				15	1	86
Peppers, hot, red, without seeds, dried (ground chili powder, added seasonings)..........1 tablespoon	15	8	2				50	2	8
Peppers, sweet:									
Raw, medium, about 6 per pound:									
Green pod without stem and seeds....1 pod	62	3	trace				15	1	93
Red pod without stem and seeds....1 pod	60	4	trace				20	1	91

NUTRITIVE VALUES OF THE EDIBLE PART OF FOOD

Food, approximate measure, and weight (in grams)		Carbo-hydrate	Fat (total lipid)	Fatty Acids			Food Energy	Pro-tein	Water
				Satu-rated (total)	Unsaturated Oleic	Unsaturated Lino-leic			
	grams	grams	grams	grams	grams	grams	Calo-ries	grams	Per-cent
Canned, pimientos, medium ....1 pod	38	2	trace				10	trace	92
Potatoes, medium (about 3 per pound raw):									
Baked, peeled after baking ....1 potato	99	21	trace				90	3	75
Boiled:									
Peeled after boiling............1 potato	136	23	trace				105	3	80
Peeled before boiling............1 potato	122	18	trace				80	2	83
French-fried, piece 2 inches by 1/2 inch by 1/2 inch:									
Cooked in deep fat ....10 pieces	57	20	7	2	2	4	155	2	45
Frozen, heated ....10 pieces	57	19	5	1	1	2	125	2	53
Mashed:									
Milk added ....1 cup	195	25	1				125	4	83
Milk and butter added ....1 cup	195	24	8	4	3	trace	185	4	80
Potato chips, medium, 2-inch diameter ....10 chips	20	10	8	2	2	4	115	1	2
Pumpkin, canned ....1 cup	228	18	1				75	2	90
Radishes, raw, small, without tops ....4 radishes	40	1	trace				5	trace	94

NUTRITIVE VALUES OF THE EDIBLE PART OF FOOD

Food, approximate measure, and weight (in grams)		Carbo-hy-drate	Fat (total lipid)	Fatty Acids			Food Energy	Pro-tein	Water
				Satu-rated (total)	Unsaturated				
					Oleic	Lino-leic			
	grams	grams	grams	grams	grams	grams	Calo-ries	grams	Per-cent
Sauerkraut, canned, solids and liquid ....1 cup	235	9	trace				45	2	93
Spinach:									
Cooked ....1 cup	180	6	1				40	5	92
Canned, drained solids ....1 cup	180	6	1				45	5	91
Canned, strained or chopped (baby food) ....1 ounce	28	2	trace				10	1	88
Sprouts, raw:									
Mung bean..........1 cup	90	6	trace				30	3	89
Soybean..........1 cup	107	4	2				40	6	89
Squash:									
Cooked:									
Summer, diced ....1 cup	210	7	trace				30	2	96
Winter, baked....1 cup	205	32	1				130	4	81
Canned, winter, strained and chopped (baby food)..........1 ounce	28	2	trace				10	trace	92
Sweet potatoes:									
Cooked, medium, 5 inches by 2 inches, weight raw about 6 ounces:									
Baked, peeled after baking.......1 sweet potato	110	36	1				155	2	64

NUTRITIVE VALUES OF THE EDIBLE PART OF FOOD

Food, approximate measure, and weight (in grams)	Carbo-hy-drate	Fat (total lipid)	Fatty Acids Saturated (total)	Unsaturated Oleic	Linoleic	Food Energy	Protein	Water
	grams	grams	grams	grams	grams	Calories	grams	Percent
grams								
Boiled, peeled after								
boiling....1 sweet potato... 147	39	1				170	2	71
Candied, 3 1/2 inches by 4 1/4 inches....1 sweet potato... 175	60	6	2	3	1	295	2	60
Canned, vacuum or solid pack....1 cup... 218	54	trace				235	4	72
Tomatoes:								
Raw, medium, 2 inches by 2 1/2 inches, about 3 per pound....1 tomato... 150	7	trace				35	2	94
Canned....1 cup... 242	10	trace				50	2	94
Tomato juice, canned....1 cup... 242	10	trace				45	2	94
Tomato catsup....1 tablespoon... 17	4	trace				15	trace	69
Turnips, cooked, diced....1 cup... 155	8	trace				35	1	94
Turnip greens: Cooked:								
In small amount of water, short time....1 cup... 145	5	trace				30	3	93
In large amount of water, long time....1 cup... 145	5	trace				25	3	94
Canned, solids and liquid....1 cup... 232	7	1				40	3	93

NUTRITIVE VALUES OF THE EDIBLE PART OF FOOD

Food, approximate measure, and weight (in grams)	Carbo-hy-drate	Fat (total lipid)	Fatty Acids			Food Energy	Pro-tein	Water
			Satu-rated (total)	Unsaturated Oleic	Lino-leic			
grams	grams	grams	grams	grams	grams	Calo-ries	grams	Per-cent
MISCELLANEOUS ITEMS								
Beer (average 3.6% alcohol by weight)............1 cup 240	9	0				100	1	92
Beverages, carbonated:								
Cola type............1 cup 240	24	0				95	0	90
Ginger ale............1 cup 230	18	0				70	0	92
Bouillon cube, 5/8 inch............1 cube 4	trace	trace				5	1	4
Chili powder. SEE Vegetables, peppers.								
Chili sauce (mainly tomatoes)............1 tablespoon 17	4	trace				20	trace	68
Chocolate:								
Bitter or baking......1 ounce 28	8	15	8	6	trace	145	3	2
Sweet............1 ounce 28	16	10	6	4	trace	150	1	1
Cider. SEE Fruits, apple juice.								
Gelatin, dry:								
Plain............1 tablespoon 10	......	trace				35	9	13
Dessert powder, 3-ounce package......1/2 cup 85	75	0				315	8	2
Gelatin dessert, ready-to-eat:								
Plain............1 cup 239	34	0				140	4	84
With fruit............1 cup 241	40	trace				160	3	82
Olives, pickled:								
Green............4 medium or 3 extra or 2 giant.. 16	trace	2	trace	2	trace	15	trace	78

NUTRITIVE VALUES OF THE EDIBLE PART OF FOOD

Food, approximate measure, and weight (in grams)		Carbohydrate	Fat (total lipid)	Fatty Acids			Food Energy	Protein	Water
				Saturated (total)	Unsaturated Oleic	Unsaturated Linoleic			
	grams	grams	grams	grams	grams	grams	Calories	grams	Percent
Ripe: Mission.......3 small or 2 large	10	trace	2	trace	2	trace	15	trace	73
Pickles, cucumber:									
Dill, large, 4 inches by 1 3/4 inches...............1 pickle	135	3	trace				15	1	93
Sweet, 2 3/4 inches by 3/4 inch..............1 pickle	20	7	trace				30	trace	61
Popcorn. SEE Grain products.									
Sherbet, orange ....1 cup	193	59	2				260	2	67
Soups, canned; ready-to-serve (prepared with equal volume of water):									
Bean with pork ...1 cup	250	22	6	1	2	2	170	8	84
Beef noodle.......1 cup	250	7	3	1	1	1	70	4	93
Beef bouillon, broth, consommé.1 cup	240	3	0	0	0	0	30	5	96
Chicken noodle...1 cup	250	8	2	trace	1	1	65	4	93
Clam chowder....1 cup	255	13	3				85	2	92
Cream soup (mushroom) ....1 cup	240	10	10	1	3	5	135	2	90
Minestrone.......1 cup	245	14	3				105	5	90

NUTRITIVE VALUES OF THE EDIBLE PART OF FOOD

Food, approximate measure, and weight (in grams)		Carbo-hy-drate	Fat (total lipid)	Fatty Acids Saturated (total)	Unsaturated Oleic	Linoleic	Food Energy	Protein	Water
	grams	grams	grams	grams	grams	grams	Calories	grams	Percent
Pea, green........1 cup	245	23	2	1	1	trace	130	6	86
Tomato........1 cup	245	16	2	trace	1	1	90	2	90
Vegetable with beef broth........1 cup	250	14	2				80	3	92
Starch (cornstarch)........1 cup	128	112	trace				465	trace	12
........1 tablespoon	8	7	trace				30	trace	12
Tapioca, quick-cooking granulated, dry, stirred before measuring........1 cup	152	131	trace				535	1	13
........1 tablespoon	10	9	trace				35	trace	13
Vinegar........1 tablespoon	15	1					2	0	....
White sauce, medium........1 cup	265	23	33	18	11	1	430	10	73
Yeast: Baker's: Compressed........1 ounce	28	3	trace				25	3	71
Dry active........1 ounce	28	11	trace				80	10	5
Brewer's, dry, debittered........1 tablespoon	8	3	trace				25	3	5
Yogurt, SEE Milk, cream, cheese: related products.									

YIELD OF COOKED MEAT PER POUND OF RAW MEAT

Meat as purchased	Meat after cooking (less drippings)	
	Parts weighed	Approximate weight of cooked parts per pound of raw meat purchased
		Ounces
Chops or steaks for broiling or frying:		
With bone and relatively large amount of fat, such as pork or lamb chops; beef rib, sirloin, or porterhouse steaks	Lean, bone, fat Lean and fat Lean only	10-12 7-10 5-7
Without bone and with very little fat, such as round of beef, veal steaks	Lean and fat Lean only	12-13 9-12
Ground meat for broiling or frying, such as hamburger, lamb, or pork patties	Patties	9-13
Roasts for oven cooking (no liquid added):		
With bone and relatively large amount of fat, such as beef rib, loin, chuck; lamb shoulder, leg; pork, fresh or cured	Lean, bone, fat Lean and fat Lean only	10-12 8-10 6-9
Without bone	Lean and fat Lean only	10-12 7-10
Cuts for pot-roasting, simmering, braising, stewing:		
With bone and relatively large amount of fat such as beef chuck, pork shoulder	Lean, bone, fat Lean and fat Lean only	10-11 8-9 6-8
Without bone and with relatively small amount of fat, such as trimmed beef, veal	Lean with adhering fat	9-11

INDEX

Raisins
  Banana Raisin Cake, 133
  Easy Raisin Bread, 109
  Raisin Bread, 115

Raspberry(ies)
  Raspberry Rhubarb Salad, 47
  Ruth's Raspberry Jam, 173

Rhubarb
  Raspberry Rhubarb Salad, 47

Rice
  Chicken Delight, 87
  Crab, Shrimp, Rice Supreme, 72
  Rice Flour Cookies, 152
  Shrimp and Rice, 72
  Super Rice, 108

Salad Dressings
  Bleu Cheese Topping, 59
  Chutney and Curry Mayonnaise, 58
  Dottie's French Dressing, 59
  Dressing à la Blanche, 57
  Easy Salad Dressing, 55
  French Vinegar Style Dressing, 58
  Fruit Dressing, 57
  Fruit Salad Dressing, 55
  Ginny's Salad Dressing, 58
  Gourmet Sour Cream Dressing, 57
  Louise's Salad Dressing, 57
  Low-Calorie Dressing, 56
  Luau Mayonnaise, 59
  Marge's Salad Dressing, 56
  Salad Dressing, 58
  Sally's Salad Dressing, 56
  Skim Milk Dressing, 56
  Thousand Island Dressing, 59
  Vinegar Dressing, 55

Salads
  Ann's Apple Salad, 50
  Apple-Celery-Cranberry-Nut Mold, 48
  Caesar Salad, 53
  Carrot Slices, 48
  Cucumber-Pineapple-Gelatin Salad, 47
  Cucumber Salad, Sweet and Sour, 45

Fish and Potato Salad, 54
Frozen Orange Fruit Salad, 51
Golden Glow Salad, 48
Hot Potato Salad, 52
Jellied Applesauce Salad, 49
Jellied Fruit Salad, 50
Laura's Jellied Vegetable Salad, 47
Lottie's Cottage Cheese Mold, 54
Margaret's Gelatin with Fruit, 51
Marinated Vegetable Toss, 45
Meat or Seafood Salad, 52
Molded Beet-Onion Salad, 50
Molded Vegetable Salad, 46
Mother's Raw Spinach Salad, 52
Nut and Cheese Salad, 54
Peach-y Salad, 49
Pepper Slaw, 46
Radish Celery Salad, 46
Raspberry Rhubarb Salad, 47
Seafood Salad, 53
Slaw, 50
Super Salad, 49
Sweet and Sour Beets, 45
Tomato and Herb Salad, 46

Salmon
  Salmon (or Tuna) Casserole, 73
  Tuna (or Salmon) Pie with Crust, 72

Sauces
  Apple Cranberry Relish, 95
  Barbecue Sauce, 92
  Barb's Barbecue Sauce, 90
  Berry Sauce, 89
  Catsup, 90
  Celery and Tomato Sauce, 94
  Cherry Glaze, 96
  Chinese Mustard, 94
  Chocolate Sauce, 99
  Citrus Fruit Sauce, 98
  Cold Shoyu (Soy) Sauce, 92
  Cream Sauce, 98
  Custard Sauce, 96
  Custard Sauce, for Shortcakes, 95
  Golden Shoyu Dip, 30
  Gravies and Approximate Exchanges, 89
  Gravy, 91
  Hawaiian Curry Sauce, 99